BIOMEDICAL ETHICS PERSPECTIVES IN THE INDIAN CONTEXT

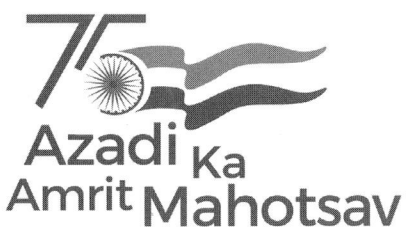

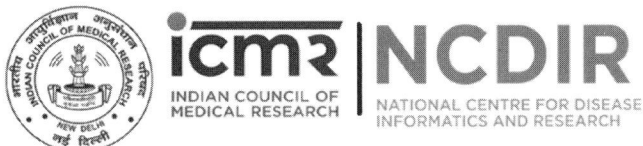

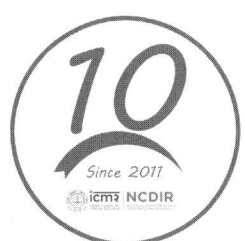

BIOMEDICAL ETHICS PERSPECTIVES IN THE INDIAN CONTEXT

Volume 1

Foreword
Balram Bhargava
Secretary to the Government of India
Department of Health Research
Ministry of Health & Family Welfare &
Director-General, ICMR

Editors
Roli Mathur
Scientist F and Head
ICMR Bioethics Unit,
National Centre for Disease Informatics and Research
(Indian Council of Medical Research)
Bengaluru, Karnataka, India

Vasantha Muthuswamy
President
Forum for Ethics Review Committees in India (FERCI)
Mumbai, Maharashtra, India

Nandini K Kumar
Vice President
Forum for Ethics Review Committees in India (FERCI)
Mumbai, Maharashtra, India

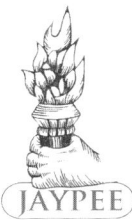

JAYPEE BROTHERS MEDICAL PUBLISHERS
The Health Sciences Publisher
New Delhi | London

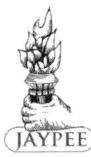 **Jaypee Brothers Medical Publishers (P) Ltd.**

Headquarters
Jaypee Brothers Medical Publishers (P) Ltd
EMCA House, 23/23-B, Ansari Road, Daryaganj
New Delhi 110 002, India
Landline: +91-11-23272143, +91-11-23272703
+91-11-23282021, +91-11-23245672
Email: jaypee@jaypeebrothers.com

Corporate Office
Jaypee Brothers Medical Publishers (P) Ltd
4838/24, Ansari Road, Daryaganj
New Delhi 110 002, India
Phone: +91-11-43574357
Fax: +91-11-43574314
Email: jaypee@jaypeebrothers.com

Overseas Office
J.P. Medical Ltd
83 Victoria Street, London
SW1H 0HW (UK)
Phone: +44 20 3170 8910
Fax: +44 (0)20 3008 6180
Email: info@jpmedpub.com

Website: www.jaypeebrothers.com
Website: www.jaypeedigital.com

© 2022, Jaypee Brothers Medical Publishers

The views and opinions expressed in this book are solely those of the original contributor(s)/author(s) and do not necessarily represent those of editor(s) of the book.

All rights reserved. No part of this publication may be reproduced, stored or transmitted in any form or by any means, electronic, mechanical, photocopying, recording or otherwise, without the prior permission in writing of the publishers.

All brand names and product names used in this book are trade names, service marks, trademarks or registered trademarks of their respective owners. The publisher is not associated with any product or vendor mentioned in this book.

Medical knowledge and practice change constantly. This book is designed to provide accurate, authoritative information about the subject matter in question. However, readers are advised to check the most current information available on procedures included and check information from the manufacturer of each product to be administered, to verify the recommended dose, formula, method and duration of administration, adverse effects and contraindications. It is the responsibility of the practitioner to take all appropriate safety precautions. Neither the publisher nor the author(s)/editor(s) assume any liability for any injury and/or damage to persons or property arising from or related to use of material in this book.

This book is sold on the understanding that the publisher is not engaged in providing professional medical services. If such advice or services are required, the services of a competent medical professional should be sought.

Every effort has been made where necessary to contact holders of copyright to obtain permission to reproduce copyright material. If any have been inadvertently overlooked, the publisher will be pleased to make the necessary arrangements at the first opportunity. The **CD/DVD-ROM** (if any) provided in the sealed envelope with this book is complimentary and free of cost. **Not meant for sale.**

Inquiries for bulk sales may be solicited at: jaypee@jaypeebrothers.com

Biomedical Ethics Perspectives in the Indian Context (Volume 1)

First Edition: **2022**

ISBN: 978-93-5465-502-9

Printed at Rajkamal Electric Press, Kundli, Haryana.

Contributors

Himanshi Chaudhary
Assistant Professor
Department of Clinical Immunology and Rheumatology
Bharati Vidyapeeth Medical College
Pune, Maharashtra, India

Mukesh Kumar
Scientist G and Head
International Health Division (IHD)
Indian Council of Medical Research (ICMR)
Headquarters
New Delhi, India

Nandini K Kumar
Vice President
Forum for Ethics Review Committees in India (FERCI)
Mumbai, Maharashtra, India

Narendra K Arora
Executive Director
INCLEN Trust International (International Clinical Epidemiology Network)
New Delhi, India

Naveen Sankhyan
Additional Professor
Department of Pediatrics
Post Graduate Institute of Medical Education and Research (PGIMER)
Chandigarh, India

Nayan Chaudhari
Assistant Professor
Department of Clinical Pharmacology
Seth GS Medical College and KEM Hospital
Mumbai, Maharashtra, India

Pandiyan Natarajan
Professor, Head and Chief Consultant
Department of Andrology and Reproductive Medicine
Chettinad Super Speciality Hospital
Chennai, Tamil Nadu, India

Pradeep Dua
Scientist C
Bureau of Indian Standards (BIS)-Headquarters, on deputation Central Council for Research in Ayurvedic Sciences (CCRAS), Ministry of Health
New Delhi, India

Prashant Mathur
Scientist G and Director
National Centre for Disease Informatics and Research (Indian Council of Medical Research)
Bengaluru, Karnataka, India

Puvithra Thanikachalam
Assistant Professor and Consultant
Department of Andrology and Reproductive Medicine
Chettinad Super Speciality Hospital
Chennai, Tamil Nadu, India

Radha Pandiyan
Associate Professor and Senior Consultant
Department of Andrology and Reproductive Medicine
Chettinad Super Speciality Hospital
Chennai, Tamil Nadu, India

Sujata Mohanty
Professor
Centre of Excellence for Stem Cell Research
All India Institute of Medical Sciences (AIIMS)
New Delhi, India

Sunita Simon Kurpad
Professor
Department of Psychiatry
Professor and Head
Department of Medical Ethics
St John's Medical College and Hospital
Bengaluru, Karnataka, India

Suvasini Sharma
Associate Professor
Department of Pediatrics
Lady Hardinge Medical College
New Delhi, India

Tulika Seth
Professor
Department of Hematology
All India Institute of Medical Sciences (AIIMS)
New Delhi, India

Urmila Thatte
Secretary
Forum for Ethics Review Committees in India (FERCI)
Mumbai, Maharashtra, India

Vasantha Muthuswamy
President
Forum for Ethics Review Committees in India (FERCI)
Mumbai, Maharashtra, India

Yashashri Shetty
Associate Professor
Department of Pharmacology and Therapeutics
Seth GS Medical College and KEM Hospital
Mumbai, Maharashtra, India

Foreword

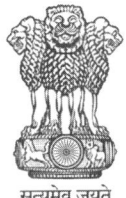

प्रोफेसर (डा.) बलराम भार्गव, पदम श्री
एमडी, डीएम, एफआरसीपी (जी.), एफआरसीपी (ई.), एफएसीसी,
एफएएचए, एफएएमएस, एफएनएएस, एफएएससी, एफ.एन.ए., डी.एस.सी.
सचिव, भारत सरकार
स्वास्थ्य अनुसंधान विभाग
स्वास्थ्य एवं परिवार कल्याण मंत्रालय एवं
महानिदेशक, आई सी एम आर

Prof. (Dr.) Balram Bhargava, Padma Shri
MD, DM, FRCP (Glasg.), FRCP (Edin.),
FACC, FAHA, FAMS, FNASc, FASc, FNA, DSc
Secretary to the Government of India
Department of Health Research
Ministry of Health & Family Welfare &
Director-General, ICMR

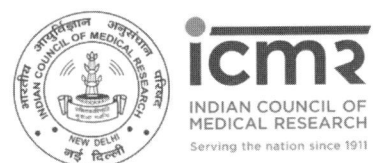

भारतीय आयुर्विज्ञान अनुसंधान परिषद
स्वास्थ्य अनुसंधान विभाग
स्वास्थ्य एवं परिवार कल्याण मंत्रालय
भारत सरकार
वी. रामलिंगस्वामी भवन, अंसारी नगर
नई दिल्ली - 110 029

Indian Council of Medical Research
Department of Health Research
Ministry of Health & Family Welfare
Government of India
V. Ramalingaswami Bhawan, Ansari Nagar
New Delhi - 110 029

I am delighted to write a foreword to the first volume of the book on "Biomedical Ethics Perspectives in the Indian Context" prepared by the ICMR Bioethics Unit, Bengaluru, Karnataka, India. The Indian Council for Medical Research (ICMR) has always been at the forefront in developing ethical guidance documents for the conduct of biomedical and health Research in India since 1980. The recent version of National Ethical Guidelines for Biomedical and Health Research Involving Human Participants, 2017 as well as the National Guidelines for Ethics Committees reviewing Biomedical and Health Research during COVID-19 Pandemic, 2020 have been recognized as a benchmark for many countries across the globe.

A multi-authored reference book covering important aspects of biomedical ethics is much needed for the different stakeholders, and this is the first of its kind in the country. This book while balancing the understanding of ethical considerations in practice and research in biomedical sciences will hopefully be useful to not only students and researchers but also ethics committee members.

I am happy to note that the editors and the authors have immensely contributed to the identified topics bringing forth the current national and international status of the ethical dilemmas and the possible solutions that could be offered to deal with them. As this book is a culmination of years of work that ICMR has done, I hope this is widely referred to across the country as guidance to encourage all researchers and other stakeholders to systematically pursue and promote fair and equitable ethical biomedical and health research.

Balram Bhargava

Preface

It gives us immense pleasure to present the ICMR Reference book on Bioethics entitled "Biomedical Ethics Perspectives in the Indian Context" to all the stakeholders in biomedical and health research in the country. The book is an endeavor to understand and tackle various ethical dilemmas arising in medical research and practice, and to guide the conduct and review of biomedical and health research. It will be the first-of-its-kind book in India compiling chapters written by multi-authors addressing the current status of ethical issues in various aspects of biomedical research and practice. We plan to bring out more such volumes in the near future.

It is expected that this would be useful in serving the needs of every biomedical and health researcher, student, or ethics committee member, providing them the ability to recognize the ethical challenges associated with research and to manage them efficiently. It would also serve as an invaluable tool to educators of bioethics as guidance to explore the ethical issues in research.

The voyage from collation and preparation of the content of the first volume of this book till its publication has been worthwhile, as it was supported by authors and reviewers, who are the very best in the field and contributed enormously to this effort. This book covers exhaustive and in-depth literature on topics like Bioethics: History and Evolution of Codes and Guidelines; Informed Consent Process; Ethics of Research Involving Children; Ethical Issues in Epidemiological Studies; Research Ethics in Participants with Mental Illness; Ethics of International Collaboration in Biomedical and Health Research: An Indian Perspective; Ethical Issues in Assisted Reproductive Technologies; Status of Traditional Medicine: Integrative and Ethical Perspectives in India, Ethical Considerations in Organ and Tissue Transplantation; and Ethical Practices and Guidelines for Animal Experimentation in Biomedical Research. Each of the chapters has been written by experts to fit the current sociocultural requirements including COVID-19 Pandemic situation and related national guidelines and regulations wherever applicable.

We, the editors, hope that the book would kindle the interest of the readers in recognizing the importance of adopting responsible ethical conduct of research and practice for protecting the rights, safety and welfare of the humanity at large.

Roli Mathur   **Vasantha Muthuswamy**   **Nandini K Kumar**

Acknowledgments

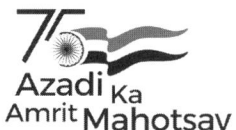

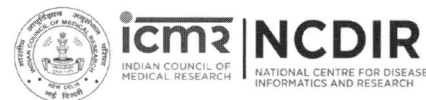

ICMR - National Centre for Disease Informatics and Research
Department of Health Research, Ministry of Health
and Family Welfare, Government of India

The book "Biomedical Ethics Perspectives in the Indian Context" is a unique contribution towards strengthening the ethical conduct of biomedical and health research in India. It has brought in inputs from several experts whose experience and knowledge has enriched it.

We express our sincere gratitude to Professor Balram Bhargava, Secretary, Department of Health Research (DHR) and Director General, Indian Council of Medical Research (ICMR) for his patronage and encouragement for the successful publication of this Reference Book.

The valuable contributions and vital efforts of the Editorial Team Members, Dr Vasantha Muthuswamy and Dr Nandini K Kumar are gratefully acknowledged. The editors identified the team of subject experts to author the chapters and closely reviewed and refined the chapters. Special thanks are due to all the authors who contributed the chapters on specialized topics sharing their expertise and knowledge. Their time and efforts are deeply acknowledged. We are immensely grateful to the peer reviewers for all the 10 chapters who provided their valuable comments for improvement.

We appreciate Mr Rajagopal Seetharaman for his efforts in copyediting the chapters, Ms Shruti Anurag Sharma for designing the cover page and the entire team at M/s Jaypee Brothers Medical Publishers (P) Ltd, New Delhi, India, for bringing this book together.

The very motivated team of scientists at ICMR Bioethics Unit, Bengaluru, Karnataka, India, especially Dr Manikandan S for his assistance during the publication stage and Dr Krupa NC and Dr Shilpi Sharma for coordinating communications and follow-ups throughout the process of compilation of chapters. The administrative support from Mr NM Ramesha, Administrative Officer along with his team from admin and finance is duly acknowledged.

It is our wish that this book will be able to serve as a teaching and training tool for students, researchers as well as members of ethics committees, and as a functional comprehensive reference material to guide the ethical conduct of biomedical and health research in India.

Roli Mathur

Prashant Mathur

About the Editors and Contributors

Editors

Roli Mathur is the Scientist F and Head of the ICMR Bioethics Unit at ICMR-NCDIR, which is also a WHO Collaborating Centre for Strengthening Ethics in Biomedical and Health Research. She is the Member Secretary of the ICMR Central Ethics Committee of Human Research (ICMR-CECHR) and the Scientific Advisor for the DHR National Ethics Committee Registry. She has coordinated the publication of various ICMR policy/guidance documents such as the National Ethical Guidelines for Biomedical Research on Human Participants (2017), the National Guidelines for Ethics Committees Reviewing Biomedical and Health Research during COVID-19 pandemic (2020), Policy on Do Not Attempt Resuscitation (2019), Common Forms for Ethics Committees (2018), etc.

Vasantha Muthuswamy is formerly Senior Deputy Director General and Head of the Division of Basic Medical Sciences including Traditional Medicine, Bioethics, and Division of Reproductive Health and Nutrition at ICMR Headquarters, New Delhi, India. She is well recognized for bringing out the ICMR Ethical Guidelines in 2000 and its subsequent revisions. She has played an active role in various national and international committees on developing ethics-related guidelines. She is the Founder Secretary of the Forum for Ethics Review Committees in Asia Pacific (FERCAP) and President of the Forum for Ethics Review Committees in India (FERCI). She currently serves as the Chairperson of the Central Ethics Committee of Human Research (ICMR-CECHR). She is internationally recognized for her leadership in research ethics and has received many Lifetime Achievement Awards.

Nandini K Kumar retired as Deputy Director General Senior Grade from ICMR, New Delhi, India. Her primary areas of expertise include Traditional Medicine Research and Bioethics. She was Fogarty Fellow Postgraduate in Bioethics from the University of Toronto and has been a member of several national and international working groups on ethics. Presently, she is the Vice President of Forum for Ethics Review Committees in India (FERCI) and Steering Committee Member of FERCAP. She was instrumental in promoting ICMR's initiatives in bioethics education in India and was closely associated in the formulation of ICMR's ethical guidelines involving human research. She is involved in numerous national and international training activities on ethical issues in biomedical and health research and traditional medicine research.

Contributors

Himanshi Chaudhary is an Assistant Professor at the Department of Clinical Immunology and Rheumatology, Bharati Vidyapeeth Medical College, Pune, Maharashtra, India.

Mukesh Kumar is currently the Head of International Health Division (IHD)-Indian Council of Medical Research (ICMR) Headquarters, New Delhi, India. He has vast experience of co-ordinating and supervising international collaboration for more than three decades. He served as the Director of Indo-French Centre for the Promotion of Advanced Research (IFCPAR/CEFIPRA) for three years. He is the Member Secretary for Health Ministry's Screening Committee (HMSC).

Narendra K Arora is the Executive Director of the INCLEN Trust International (International Clinical Epidemiology Network) and the President of Institute Body at All India Institute of Medical Sciences (AIIMS), Patna and Deoghar. He retired as Professor of Pediatric Gastroenterology, Hepatology and Nutrition from AIIMS, New Delhi, India. He is a well-known Public Health Expert involved in policy making, program planning, implementation and evaluation of public health programmes at national and international level.

Naveen Sankhyan is an Additional Professor at the Department of Pediatrics, Post Graduate Institute of Medical Education and Research (PGIMER), Chandigarh, India. He has contributed to more than 35 chapters in various textbooks and has numerous publications in various national and international indexed journals.

Nayan Chaudhari is an Assistant Professor at the Department of Clinical Pharmacology, Seth GS Medical College and KEM Hospital, Mumbai, Maharashtra, India. He has several publications to his credit in good peer-reviewed journals.

Pandiyan Natarajan is the Professor and Head at the Department of Andrology and Reproductive Medicine, Chettinad Super Speciality Hospital, Chennai, Tamil Nadu, India. He is a Pioneer in the field of Human Reproduction in South India and one among very few in India, popular teacher, trainer, researcher of national and international reputation and thrice awardee of Lifetime Achievement Awards. Many of his publications in national, international journals and books reflect his innovative thinking and challenges in the practice of male and female infertility.

Pradeep Dua is currently working as Research Officer, Drugs Control Cell, Ministry of AYUSH, New Delhi. He has earned professional qualifications in the fields of Hospital Management, Intellectual Property Rights Law, Bioethics, Pharmaceutical Drugs Regulatory Affairs, Clinical Research, Yoga, and Naturopathy.

Prashant Mathur is the Director of ICMR-NCDIR, Bengaluru, Karnataka, India, and is a Pediatrician experienced in working on several research study designs and multi-centric epidemiology projects. His current focus of work is on Epidemiology of Noncommunicable Diseases (NCDs), Disease registries and Surveillance of NCDs.

Puvithra Thanikachalam is an Assistant Professor at the Department of Andrology and Reproductive Medicine, Chettinad Super Speciality Hospital, Chennai, Tamil Nadu, India, and Editor in the Chettinad Health City Medical Journal. She is a passionate teacher and awarded for academic excellence.

Radha Pandiyan is an Associate Professor and Senior Consultant at the Department of Andrology and Reproductive Medicine, Chettinad Super Speciality Hospital, Chennai, Tamil Nadu, India. She is a passionate teacher and trainer. She has been in the field of Human Reproduction for 30 years and played key roles in many national and international contributions by the team. She initiated the unique annual follow-up of children born after assisted conception, which completed 10 years.

Sujata Mohanty is presently working as a Professor in the Centre of Excellence for Stem Cell Research, All India Institute of Medical Sciences (AIIMS), New Delhi, India. She initiated basic research using adult, Embryonic and Induced Pluripotent Stem Cells for a better understanding of Stem Cell Biology and Drug Discovery at AIIMS. She is the Chairperson and Member of Institutional Committee for Stem Cell Research (ICSCR) of 12 Institutions in the country.

Sunita Simon Kurpad is currently the Professor, Department of Psychiatry, and Professor and Head, Department of Medical Ethics at St John's Medical College and Hospital, Bengaluru, Karnataka, India. She has been working as a Faculty Member at St John's Medical College and Hospital, Bengaluru, for the last 25 years.

Suvasini Sharma is an Associate Professor at the Department of Pediatrics, Lady Hardinge Medical College (LHMC), New Delhi, India. She is the Member Secretary of the Research and Project Committee, LHMC and Smt Sucheta Kriplani Hospital, New Delhi.

Tulika Seth is a Professor at the Department of Hematology, All India Institute of Medical Sciences (AIIMS), New Delhi, India. She has conducted more than 200 allogeneic hematopoietic stem cell transplants and executed the first umbilical cord blood transplant as well as the first transplant for multiple sclerosis (MS) and the first haplo-transplant in the Department of Hematology at AIIMS. She has authored more than 150 papers and over 40 book chapters.

Urmila Thatte is an Emeritus Professor at Seth GS Medical College and KEM Hospital, Mumbai, Maharashtra, India, after serving there as Professor and Head at the Department of Clinical Pharmacology for several years. She is the Secretary of the Forum for Ethics Review Committees in India (FERCI), Mumbai. She was the Member of the core team that wrote the ICMR Bioethics Guidelines.

Yashashri Shetty is working as an Associate Professor in the Department of Pharmacology and Therapeutics at Seth GS Medical College and KEM Hospital, Mumbai, Maharashtra, India. She has been associated with the Ethics Committee functioning for the last 15 years.

Contents

1. Bioethics: History and Evolution of Codes and Guidelines 1
Vasantha Muthuswamy
- Bioethics *2*
- Biomedical Research Ethics *2*
- Basic Principles and Guidelines *2*
- Bioethics Education and Training *10*

2. Informed Consent Process 13
Urmila Thatte, Yashashri Shetty, Nayan Chaudhari
- Guidelines and Regulations *13*
- Stakeholders in the Informed Consent Process *15*
- Components of the Informed Consent Document *15*
- Considerations in Administration and Documentation of Consent *16*
- Types of Consent (Written, Oral, Audio, AV, Electronic, Reconsent, Tiered Consent, Broad, Specific, Implied, etc.) *18*
- Consent from Vulnerable Groups: Assent and Parental/LAR Consent in Children *19*
- Informed Consent Review: Roles of Ethics Committee Members *20*
- Future Requirements *21*

3. Ethics of Research Involving Children 23
Himanshi Chaudhary, Suvasini Sharma, Naveen Sankhyan
- Why Research Involving Children? *24*
- Unique Challenges in Children *24*
- Challenges in the Developing World *25*
- Issue of Assent/Consent *26*
- Protection of the Interests of the Child *27*
- Research in Special Situations *27*

4. Ethical Issues in Epidemiological Studies 30
Prashant Mathur, Narendra K Arora
- Epidemiological Study Methods *30*
- Ethical Contexts in Epidemiological Research *31*
- Specific Issues in Epidemiological Research *31*

5. Research Ethics in Participants with Mental Illness 42
Sunita Simon Kurpad
- The Role of Nature of Illness, its Course, and Setting of Research *42*
- The Three Central Areas of Vulnerability *43*
- Arenas of Ethical Concerns *43*

6. Ethics of International Collaboration in Biomedical and Health Research: An Indian Perspective 52
Mukesh Kumar
- Modes of International Collaboration *53*
- Collaborative Research in Health Sciences *53*
- Role and Composition of Health Ministry's Screening Committee *54*
- Ethics of International Collaboration *54*
- Role of Ethics Committees *55*
- Concerns on Ethical Issues and HMSC Submission *55*
- Some Practical Illustrations on Working of EC *57*

7. Ethical Issues in Assisted Reproductive Technologies ... 59
Puvithra Thanikachalam, Radha Pandiyan, Pandiyan Natarajan
- Reproduction: A Fundamental Right *59*
- Assisted Reproductive Technologies *59*
- The Embryo *61*
- Third-party Reproduction *62*
- Uterine Transplantation *64*
- Designer Babies *64*
- Posthumous Collection of Gametes *64*
- Religious Issues in Assisted Reproductive Technology *64*
- Ethical Issues in Assisted Reproductive Technology *64*
- ICMR Guidelines and the ART Regulations Bill *65*

8. Status of Traditional Medicine: Integrative and Ethical Perspectives in India ... 67
Nandini K Kumar, Pradeep Dua
- Status of Traditional Indian Medicine in India *69*
- Funding for Research on Traditional Medicine *70*
- Medical Ethics in Indian Systems of Medicine *70*
- Ethical Guidelines and Regulations *70*
- Research in India *72*
- Integrative Initiatives *72*
- Chemical-Manufacturing-Control *73*
- Nonclinical Studies *74*
- Clinical Studies *74*
- Ethical Issues *75*

9. Ethical Considerations in Organ and Tissue Transplantation ... 79
Tulika Seth, Sujata Mohanty
- Hematopoietic Stem Cell Transplantation *79*
- Solid Organ and Tissue Transplantation *84*
- Other New Types of Transplants *90*

10. Ethical Practices and Guidelines for Animal Experimentation in Biomedical Research ... 94
Vasantha Muthuswamy
- Historical Perspective *94*
- Controversies in Animal Experimentation: The Never-ending Debate *94*
- Emergence of Animal Ethical Guidelines: An Indian Perspective *95*
- Significance of Animals in Biomedical Research *97*
- Animal Species Used in Biomedical Research *98*
- Ethics of Animal Experimentation and the Development of "Rs" *98*
- Constitution of Institutional Animal Ethics Committee *99*
- Functions of Animal Ethics Committee *100*

Index ... *103*

Bioethics: History and Evolution of Codes and Guidelines

Vasantha Muthuswamy

ABSTRACT

Ethics refers to the moral code of conduct that is to be followed by a civil society. Bioethics or biomedical ethics relates to the moral problems arising in the practice of medicine and the pursuit of biomedical research. It is the study of the ethical issues emerging from advances in biology and medicine and examines the relationships among life sciences, biotechnology, medicine and medical ethics, philosophy, law, theology, sociology, and health policy. The ethical code of conduct for physicians, which existed from ancient times, has undergone innumerable changes over a period of time due to advances in biomedicine and emerging new technologies as well as concept of morality and its varied interpretation by different disciplines of art and science. The evolution of modern bioethics in the 20th century following unethical practices in health care and medical research led to the development of various codes, guidelines, and regulations by individual countries as well as global organizations. This is an emerging dynamic area undergoing constant changes requiring continuous training of all the stakeholders involved in health care and biomedical research. Bioethics contributes to the rights of patients and research participants as autonomous persons who should be protected at all times and responsibilities of healthcare professionals and researchers. Although the ethical theories may differ, the four basic principles that should be adhered to are nonmaleficence, beneficence, respect for individual autonomy, and justice. The evolution of the codes and guidelines and its applications will be examined from the international and national perspectives emphasizing the need for bioethics education and training of all the stakeholders in India.

INTRODUCTION

Ethics is a generic term referring to the moral code of conduct in a civil society. It concerns the rules, customs, and beliefs of a society along with the scholarly efforts to articulate and analyze the same and to enable members of the society to follow the same. It is generally agreed that "morality" is the theory about right and wrong and the common morality comprises socially approved norms of human conduct, which existed even before we were instructed about its relevant rules and regulations. As we grow beyond infancy, we learn moral norms along with other social values. Later in life, we are able to distinguish between general social norms observed commonly by members of the society from specific social norms binding the members of special groups such as members of a profession. Professionals are usually identified by their commitment to provide important services to clients or consumers through specialized training. The concept of a medical professional is closely linked to a background of distinct education, knowledge, and skills, which should be morally used to benefit patients. Healthcare professions typically specify and enforce obligations, thereby seeking to ensure that persons who enter into relationships with members of the same profession will find them competent and trustworthy. Thus, a professional code represents an articulated statement of the role based on morality as professional standards for that particular profession.

The ethical codes of conduct for medical professionals and physicians existed since time immemorial, the most ancient of these being documented in Siddha (30th century BC) and Ayurveda (10th century BC to 1st and 2nd century AD). Caraka Samhita[1] of Ayurveda prescribes the duties of physicians toward their patients and other fellow professionals. A similar code also exists for surgeons in Sushruta Samhita. "Hippocratic Oath" of the Greco-Roman period is the most well-known of such codes in the Western world for modern medicine. All these and other such codes have stemmed out of the basic concept of "nonmaleficence", that is, "Do No Harm," which was the driving principle for all physicians and healthcare professionals focusing on the rights of those receiving health services and the obligations of health professionals.[2] Unani medicine of the Babylonian origin, which strongly imbibed Hippocratic tenets, also follows the same principle. Most of the medical councils around the world have prescribed codes for the medical professionals of the respective countries. The prestige the medical profession enjoys in the eyes of the society is related to its contributions to the well-being of the society and the quality of performance by its members in adhering to laid-down principles of doing no harm, relieving pain and suffering, maintaining confidentiality, and being trustworthy and fair in their dealings with the patients with whom they share a fiduciary relationship.

BIOETHICS

However, this centuries-old code of conduct for physicians was subjected to repeated challenges as newer concepts of health and healing emerged over centuries. In 1657, the concept of "just moral propriety in medicine" was propounded by Thomas Hobbes.[3] Thomas Percival came up with the concept of code of medical ethics for the first time[4] and in the 18th century that of "medical humanism" by John Gregory.[5] In 1846, the American Medical Association (AMA) brought out the first national code of medical ethics. Claude Bernard introduced the topic of "experimental medicine" in 1865 wherein he held that the individual's interest was to be considered over and above societal benefit. In 1897, the AMA revised its code.[6] As the medicine of the 19th century absorbed advances in science and technology and learned to use the numerical method of evaluating the results of treatment, knowledge and skill became more measurable. Fritz Jahr used the word "bioethics" for the first time in an article titled "Bio-Ethics: A Review of the Ethical Relationships of Humans to Animals and Plants" where he proposed a "Bioethical Imperative" for use of animals and plants by humans. In the decade during and after the two World Wars, medical sciences had advanced to such a great extent that medical interventions became increasingly technical, prompting medical ethics to a new perspective. Added to the conventional theology and philosophy, newer disciplines of law and sociology became engaged in ethical discourses of medicine and science.[7] Although Fritz was the first to use the word "bioethics," it was first coined by Van Rensselaer Potter, at the University of Wisconsin, in an article "Bioethics, the Science of Survival" and a book Bioethics: Bridge of the future (1970–71).[8] He added the biosphere to the concept while Dr Andre Hellegers developed it as a new academic topic at the Kennedy Institute for the Study of Human Reproduction and Bioethics. This was a combination of knowledge of biology and human value systems. In 1972, Warren T Reich brought out the Encyclopedia of Bioethics wherein he introduced this subject as "the study of the ethical dimensions of medicine and biological sciences."[9]

BIOMEDICAL RESEARCH ETHICS

The ancient codes of ethics directed the physicians that they have a moral obligation to attain new knowledge and skill. From the beginning of medicine, physicians knew that prior treatment success might fail in a current instance. In desperate moments of illness, previously untried remedies were attempted, sometimes with unexpected success. However, the traditional aim of "do no harm" and the Hippocratic maxim "benefit and do no harm" urged physicians to maintain a constant intent to cure. Medical history hints that certain Alexandrian physicians were permitted to perform vivisection on criminals and these experimenters were referred to as "medical murderers" by the Greek medical encyclopedist Celsus.[10] Much later in 1865, the noted French physiologist and Father of Experimental Medicine, Claude Bernard, stated, "it is our duty and right to perform experiments on man whenever it can save his life, cure him or gain him some personal benefits. The principle of medical and surgical morality, therefore, consists in never performing on man an experiment, which might be harmful to him to any extent, even though the result may be highly advantageous to science, and to the health of others".[11] Thus, one can see that while advocating experiments on fellow human beings, Bernard's principle lies within the Hippocratic tradition. The enthusiasm for experimentation grew during the 19th century and early 20th century. The worst "scientific experiments" came to light following the World War II at the doctors' trial in Nuremberg where innumerable atrocities committed by Nazi physicians on uninformed prisoners of war in the name of medical research came to light and shocked the entire world. During the Nuremberg Military Tribunal's meeting, the studies conducted by the Nazi physicians on unsuspecting prisoners of war were openly discussed. Some of the brutalities performed in the name of medical research were high-altitude experiments, freezing experiments, malaria and typhus experiments, sulfanilamide and poison experiments, phosphorous burns and chemical sterilization, and transplantation studies. The end point of many of the experiments was death. Other than these experiments, hundreds of prisoners were killed to collect skeletons for an anthropological investigation. In addition to sentencing the accused, the Military Tribunal judges articulated the proclamation of the Nuremberg Code on Experimentation in Human Subjects in 1947,[12] containing 10 principles of acceptable research involving humans, marking a new era of code of ethics for medical research, which is the most widely known document on ethics of research. This drew unprecedented attention from public, professionals, and policy makers. A new beginning was made in the moral traditions of medicine and laid the foundation for the new discipline of Biomedical Research Ethics.

BASIC PRINCIPLES AND GUIDELINES

The four cardinal virtues of a health professional are compassion, discernment, trustworthiness, and integrity. Truth telling and consent seeking have long been part of an indigenous medical tradition based on medical theories that taught that knowledge and autonomy had demonstrably beneficial effects on most patients' health. The principle of autonomy implies that physicians must inform their patients about the nature of the condition and its expected course and the benefits and risks of any proposed treatment and of alternative treatments, if available. It is also emphasized that doctors and patients should make joint decisions. Maintaining the confidentiality of patients' information is the duty of the physicians. Hence, the rights of the patients and the responsibilities of the physicians constitute the basic principles of ethics of medical practice.

The Nuremberg Code has delineated 10 basic principles for medical research that must be observed to satisfy moral, ethical, and legal concepts. Voluntary consent of the human subjects, experimental results to bring good to the society, prior experiments with animals, avoidance of unnecessary physical and mental suffering, prior assurance that no death or disability will result, the scientific qualification of researchers, evaluation by subject's rights, risks should not exceed benefits, adequate facilities to protect subjects and researcher's duty to terminate harmful experiments are the 10 principles of this Code which hold good till date. Almost two decades later, the World Medical Association at its 18th assembly brought out the Helsinki Declaration in 1964 to guide the treating physicians about the norms to be followed in therapeutic as well as nontherapeutic research.[13] However, the existence of these two codes did not guarantee strict compliance by the physicians while performing research, as revealed by a landmark article in 1966 by Dr Henry K Beecher, a professor of anesthesiology at the Harvard Medical School. Dr Beecher published the article "Ethics in Clinical Research" in the New England Journal of Medicine[14] where he described 22 studies which violated the basic norms of ethics while doing research with human beings. These experiments performed by respected investigators at leading medical institutions were published in reputed journals. Some of the examples are a research performed at the Jewish Chronic Disease Hospital in elderly patients where cancer cells were injected in those without any cancer, a study in soldiers with streptococcal throat infection who were denied treatment with Penicillin although the participants were likely to develop rheumatic heart disease, and a physiological research in which a needle was inserted into the left atrium during bronchoscopy without any benefit to the individuals. The most infamous of these studies was the Willowbrook Study in which researchers deliberately exposed children and adolescents to hepatitis virus at a New York state facility for orphans to understand the natural history of viral hepatitis. The most well-debated of these was the Tuskegee Syphilis Study in the Alabama county conducted by the United States Department of Health and Human Services (HHS), in which more than 400 African-Americans were observed for natural history of syphilis from 1932 to 1972, although Penicillin had been discovered in the early 1940s and found to be the drug of choice as a cure for syphilis. The participants were not informed about the true nature of the study and were followed for 40 years until exposed by a press reporter in 1972 when the study was forced to be stopped and a National Commission was set up to come out with a report. The commission was charged with "identifying the basic ethical principles that should underline the conduct of biomedical and behavioral research involving human subjects, and ... develop[ing] guidelines which should be followed to assure that such research is conducted in accordance with those principles." The commission identified three such basic principles as being "particularly relevant to the ethics of research involving human subjects: the principles of respect for persons (autonomy), beneficence and justice." This led to the release of the Belmont Report in 1979, which is the first national guidelines for medical research.[15] The enquiry further continued as the Tuskegee Study exemplified a pattern of institutionalized racism in health care and ultimately after 25 years of enquiry, in the year 1997, President Bill Clinton tendered a public apology and paid a compensation of 7 billion US dollars to the affected families in addition to setting up the Tuskegee University National Center for Bioethics in Research and Health. The Tuskegee Syphilis Study thus had a wider repercussion forcing the creation of the National Commission for the Protection of the Human Subjects of Biomedical and Behavioral Research as well as the enactment of an act governing research with humans in 1974 in USA.[16]

Following the formulation of the Nuremberg Code, Helsinki Declaration and Belmont Report, a number of other guidelines, declarations, codes, and reports were prepared by many national and international organizations. In 1980, the Indian Council of Medical Research issued a "Policy Statement on Ethical Considerations for Research on Human Subjects,"[17] and subsequently many other countries and international agencies released their respective guidelines. Thus, the necessity of adhering to the principles enunciated in the Nuremberg Code and Helsinki Declaration got top priority in various countries during the 1970s and 1980s and resulted in the formulation of numerous national and international guidelines to protect the individuals participating in research from any harm.

During the following decades, there was a quantitative increase in medical research but it was also accompanied by qualitative improvement in research methodologies, ethical review, and evaluation of research results. The Constitution of Ethics Committees or Institutional Review Boards became a practice, and the peer review of research was done based on the basic principles enshrined in the codes and guidelines followed by different countries. The classic textbook of bioethics followed by many across the world is that of Tom Beauchamp and James Childress (1979) entitled "Principles of Biomedical Ethics," which lays emphasis on the fact that "principles provide the most general and comprehensive norms ... that guide actions. The difference [between rules and principles] is that rules are more specific in content and more restricted in scope than principles."[18] Their approach is known as principlism, or the four-principle approach, to biomedical ethics or more light-heartedly known as the "Georgetown Mantra". Principlism is a normative ethical framework designed for decision-making in health care. It is a common morality approach relying on the following four principles and applicable in a wide variety of contexts involving clinician–patient interactions.

1. *Autonomy*: Respect for persons and right of individuals for self-determination. This principle recognizes that a patient's choice should be autonomous in nature if:
   - The choice is voluntary,
   - The patient is adequately informed, and
   - The patient possesses decision-making capacity or competence.
2. *Nonmaleficence*: This principle denotes "do no harm" and refers to the core value of medical profession.
3. *Beneficence*: This principle means fruitful result and the need to "do good." The principle of beneficence asserts:
   - The duty to help all concerned and encompasses both specific and general beneficence.
4. *Justice*: This principle pertains to selection of participants and equitable distribution of burden of risks and benefits of research. The principle of justice requires that equals be treated equally and unequals be treated in proportion to their relevant inequalities.

The text by Beauchamp and Childress is probably the most authoritative work on "principlism," and it seems that most bioethical decisions are analyzed using the framework described therein. Another popular text by the same author, "'The Four Principles' Approach to Health Care Ethics",[19] employs the same four principles as a practical approach in the practice of medicine. Beauchamp and Childress derived their principles by analyzing various ethical theories relevant to the subject of biomedical ethics, since according to them a well-developed ethical theory provides a framework within which agents can reflect on the acceptability of actions and can evaluate moral judgments and moral character. Some of the theories are indispensable for a reflective study on biomedical ethics because much of the literature draws on methods and conclusions found in these theories such as utilitarianism, Kantianism, character ethics, communitarianism, the ethics of care, and common morality accounts. The two most talked about of these are the utilitarian and Kantian theories. The utilitarian theory is a consequence-based theory according to which actions are right or wrong according to the balance of their good and bad consequences, that is, the principle of utility which asserts that we always ought to produce the maximal balance of positive value over disvalue. The Kantianism is an obligation-based theory proposed by Immanuel Kant (1724–1804) which insists on right actions in addition to consequences. This is also known as the deontological theory. This principle categorically requires that we should never treat another as a means to our ends.[20] Thus, it can be seen that both these theories express the language of obligations and rights. The discussions also draw from the other theories mentioned above, as contemporary biomedical ethics incorporates theoretical conflicts that exist among the various normative theories related to morality. Almost all ethical theories converge to the conclusion that the most important ingredient in a person's moral life is a developed character that provides the inner motivation and strength to do what is right and good.

The purpose of research, its potential benefits to participants, the anticipated risks and compensations for the same, the unexpected consequences and steps proposed to tackle the same, and the evaluation of risk–benefit ratio are all covered under the principles of Nonmaleficence and Beneficence. The fundamental moral principle of "respect for persons" demands a voluntary, informed consent from individuals participating in research and is termed the "Autonomy" principle. This includes right to privacy and confidentiality and obligations to obtain an informed consent from the legally authorized/acceptable representatives wherever necessary to protect the vulnerable groups who lack autonomy to take decisions on their own. Recruitment of those with diminished autonomy also requires special consideration and adequate justification for involving them in research. Hence, obtaining "informed consent" has become the most crucial requirement in any clinical research. Instead of treating it as a one-time activity, it is a series of continuous procedures throughout the research period because of which it is termed the informed consent process.

The principle of Justice demands that the beneficial outcome of research is equitably distributed amongst the research participants and other beneficiaries, if any. The burden of research cannot be borne by a group of individuals while the benefits of that research are enjoyed by another elite group. This has gained global importance in view of the growing international collaboration between developed and developing countries. Selection of participants and study design with equitable access to post trial benefits is the hallmark of this principle. All clinical research involving human participants are required to consider the above principles while planning, conducting, evaluating, reporting, and utilizing the research results.

The recent advances in science and technology are mind-boggling. What was considered as science fiction till recent years has now become a reality, thereby creating numerous ethical dilemmas in its wake. The unprecedented advances in modern biology, biotechnology, genetics, reproductive technologies, neurobiology, and allied fields of biomedical sciences during the last couple of decades, having immense potential for human welfare, have also created complex ethical dilemmas for both the scientists and the medical practitioners. "Some have even wondered if our scientific capabilities are matched by our ability to identify, debate, and formulate policies in respect to the impact of these discoveries on the ethical, legal, social, psychological, cultural, and economic consequences on individuals, communities, and human race in general".[21] Each of these requires careful scrutiny by appropriate scientific and ethics review committees before any research is undertaken. The controversial issues are so many and so complicated that each one of them requires closer scrutiny and consensus decision. Advances in biotechnology, genomics, genetic engineering, organ and tissue transplantation, new reproductive technologies, stem cell research including cloning, medical devices, recombinant products, surgical innovations, life support systems, all pose challenges to the conscientious researchers for which acceptable solutions need to get evolved to benefit the majority. Constant debates are the need of the hour as there is no single solution to any issue and decisions have to be taken on a case-to-case basis. This responsibility for approving any research to be undertaken is entrusted to an ethics committee (EC). It is named as Institutional Review Board (IRB)/ Ethics Committee (EC)/Research Ethics Committee (REC)/Ethics Review Committee (ERC), etc. It comprises members from different walks of life such as physicians, scientists, technologists, social scientists, philosophers, religious experts, legal personnel, and even lay persons to assess each research protocol for its scientific as well as ethical validity. The combined wisdom of all these people having different expertise will decide whether any research can be undertaken or not. This requirement was proposed by the Helsinki Declaration in 1975 resulting in many institutions in the US and Europe setting up their institutional review boards, but the details of their structure and functioning became more authoritative and streamlined after the Belmont Report and the subsequent guidelines.

International Guidelines

Declaration of Helsinki

It is interesting to take stock of how the DOH (Declaration of Helsinki) evolved over the years. The first version released by the World Medical Assembly (WMA) in 1964 at Helsinki in Finland followed the crisis in research ethics during World War II. The first revision was made in Tokyo, Japan, in 1975, which first introduced the concept of an independent committee to review research proposals. Researchers were continued to be governed by the 1975 version for the next 25 years, till the fifth version was released in Scotland in 2000.[22]

The second, third, and fourth versions were released in the intervening 25 years. There were relatively minor changes in the second revision which included consent of minors and in the third revision, improvement in structure and function of ethics committee. The fourth revision of 1996 created the controversy about use of placebos against the background of test therapies for HIV/AIDS. The fifth revision of 2000 was the most debated, challenged, and controversial version and formed the topic of seminars and conferences all over the world. The three major newly introduced topics which were the cause of all these deliberations were the use of placebos, best current therapeutic interventions as the standard-of-care comparator in the control arm, and post-trial access to proven interventions in the context of increasing international collaboration for research in HIV/AIDS. There were two corrections made related to paragraph 29 (about use of placebo) and paragraph 30 (post-trial access to best proven intervention) in 2002 and 2004, respectively. The highlights of the sixth revision in 2008 were that clinical trials registry be maintained, outcome of trials be accessible in public domain, research-related injury be compensated, and post-trial access and availability of proven therapies/diagnostics be considered. The last in the series was the seventh version released in 2013 in Brazil. Compared to the original 11 articles in the 1964 version, this version has 37, two each under the preamble (1–2), 13 articles under the General Principles (3–15), eight under informed consent (25–32), three under risk, burden and benefits (16–18), two under vulnerable groups and individuals (19–20), and two under scientific requirements and research protocol (21–22). One article each is devoted to research ethics committees, privacy and confidentiality, the use of placebo, post-trial provisions, and administration of unproven therapies.[23]

The following provisions have been introduced for the first time:
- Appropriate compensation and treatment must be ensured for those harmed in research (Articles 15 and 22).
- The researchers should undertake monitoring of the risks, assessment, and documentation (Article 17).
- After the study has been concluded, the researchers must submit to the committee a final report that contains a summary of the findings and conclusions (Article 23).
- All study subjects involved in medical research should be given the option of being informed about the general outcome and results of the study (Article 27).
- Every research study involving human subjects must be registered in a publicly accessible database (Article 35).

WHO CIOMS Guidelines

The World Health Organization (WHO) and the United Nations Educational, Scientific, and Cultural Organization (UNESCO) cooperated in 1949 to establish the Council of

International Organizations of Medical Sciences (CIOMS). The Council represents a substantial proportion of the international community of scientific organizations in biomedicine with 49 national and international organizations, such as national academies and medical research councils as members/representatives. The goals of CIOMS are, among others, to serve the scientific interests of the international biomedical community and to foster international collaborations. CIOMS published the Proposed International Guidelines for Biomedical Research Involving Human Subjects in 1982[24] in close collaboration with the WHO. These guidelines, which are still valid today, have two objectives: to apply the principles of the Declaration of Helsinki and to specify these principles in the context of international biomedical research, especially in low-resource settings. The first version of the International Guidelines for Biomedical Research Involving Human Subjects, 1993,[25] replaced the "proposed guidelines" of 1982. CIOMS updated and revised these guidelines from 1998 to 2002. The new 2002 text, which superseded that of 1993, consists of a statement of general ethical principles, a preamble and 21 guidelines, with an introduction and a brief account of earlier instruments and guidelines.[26] Like the 1982 and 1993 guidelines, this publication was also designed to be of use, particularly to low-resource countries, in defining national policies on the ethics of biomedical research, applying ethical standards in local circumstances, and establishing or redefining adequate mechanisms for ethical review of research involving human subjects. In 2010, the CIOMS executive committee decided to bring out the next revision. In September 2015, a draft of the guidelines was published and the final version of the guidelines was accepted by the General Assembly of CIOMS on November 29, 2016.[27] The CIOMS guidelines put forward fundamental justification for research such as social value, adequate risk–benefit ratio, informed consent, research in low-resource settings, research in disaster situations, and cluster randomized trials. The guidelines combine key principles with a guide to their application based on the state of the art in research ethics. In a brief overview, one may group the 25 guidelines as in **Table 1**.

The revised guidelines thus represent a timely and indispensable orientation for researchers, ethics committees, and other stakeholders in health-related research.[27]

ICH-GCP Guidelines

The ICH Harmonized Tripartite Guidelines (ICH-GCP) for Good Clinical Practice is the product of an ambitious international partnership between USA, Japan, and Europe promulgated in 1996, which gives in detail standards for ethics review committees, investigators, and sponsors. The guideline was developed by considering the current good clinical practices of the European Union, Japan, and the United States as well as those of Australia, Canada, the Nordic countries, and the WHO. This guideline was to be followed when generating clinical trial data for drugs and devices that are intended to be submitted to regulatory authorities with emphasis on protection of safety and well-being of the research subjects and production of credible data.[28] The principles established in this guideline may also be applied to other types of clinical research that may have an impact on the safety and well-being of human subjects.

TABLE 1: CIOMS guidelines and their principles.

Guidelines	Principles
Guideline 1	Lays the normative foundation of health-related research with social value and scientific validity
Guidelines 2 and 3	Extend this foundation to low-resource settings by arguing for specific aspects of justice in the distribution of social value and the fair selection of participants
Guideline 4	Gives a precise description of how an appropriate risk–benefit ratio can be determined
Guidelines 5 and 6	Contain specifications relating to risk–benefit evaluations: The choice of the control group, whether an effective established intervention exists, and the requirements of care for participants' health needs
Guidelines 7 and 8	Spell out principles for community engagement, collaborative partnership, and capacity building
Guideline 9	Is the fundamental guideline on informed consent
Guidelines 10, 11, and 12	Address specific contexts of informed consent, namely, the conditions for waivers, biobanking, and research with health data
Guideline 13	Treats general questions of reimbursement and compensation
Guideline 14	Dedicated to treatment and compensation for research-related harms
Guideline 15	Issues related to vulnerability
Guidelines 16, 17, 18, and 19	Address individuals and groups who may potentially be vulnerable in specific ways (those incapable of giving consent, children and adolescents, women, and pregnant and breastfeeding women)
Guidelines 20, 21, and 22	Deal with specific types of research, which recently became more important (research in disasters and disease outbreaks, cluster randomized trials, and the use of online environment and digital tools)
Guideline 23	Describes all the requirements for ethics review
Guidelines 24 and 25	Prescribes rules for transparency, which should contribute to meeting some of the challenges for social and scientific value (public accountability and conflicts of interest)

(CIOMS: Council of International Organizations of Medical Sciences)

Since the development of the ICH-GCP Guideline, the scale, complexity and cost of clinical trials have increased. Evolutions in technology and risk management processes offer new opportunities to increase efficiency and focus on relevant activities. When the original ICH E6 (R1) text was prepared, clinical trials were performed using a largely paper-based process. Technical advances in use of electronic data recording and reporting facilitated better data management. Therefore, this guideline has been amended in November, 2016 as E6 (R2) to encourage implementation of improved and more efficient approaches to clinical trial design, conduct, performance, oversight, auditing, recording, analysis, and reporting while continuing to ensure human subject protection and reliability of trial results. Standards regarding electronic records and essential documents intended to increase clinical trial quality and efficiency, and risk-based management mainly by the sponsors has been incorporated.[29] The use of electronic media for data management has become more advantageous in the COVID-19 pandemic scenario during 2020–21. Further discussion is ongoing with participation from many more countries (India included) for further streamlining the standards.

Nuffield Council on Bioethics

Apart from the general guidelines for medical research and clinical trials, different agencies have been bringing out specific guidelines on relevant topics. The Nuffield Council on Bioethics is a UK-based independent charitable body, which examines and reports on bioethical issues raised by new advances in biological and medical research. Established in 1991, the Council is funded by the Nuffield Foundation, the Medical Research Council, and the Wellcome Trust. The Council has been described by the media as a "leading ethics watchdog," which "never shrinks from the unthinkable." The Nuffield Council has released almost 40 guidelines since its inception on varied subjects such as human tissue, human genetics, xenotransplantation, mental health, clinical trials, international collaboration, pharmacogenetics, animal experiments, stem cell research, genetic screening, medical profiling and online medicine, DNA profiling, emerging biotechnologies, and many more including genome editing and its social and reproductive issues. The Council selects topics to examine through a horizon scanning program, which aims to identify developments relevant to biological and medical research. Generally, their recommendations are considered quite influential to policy makers.[30] During the COVID-19 pandemic, the Council brought out a number of policy briefs related to ethical, social, and policy issues to guide the researchers and the government for taking appropriate decisions.[31]

UNESCO Guidelines

UNESCO continues to play a vital role in arousing international awareness about the ethical issues (specially their impact on human rights) emerging from modern biological research. In 1989, the Director-General was invited by the General Conference "to consider ways and means of introducing a permanent system of consultation for the exchange of information and experience on the ethical implications of contemporary science and technology in order to make UNESCO a world clearing-house for information and documentation on this question at a time of decisive advances in the life sciences and, in particular in their medical applications." As a follow-up of this resolution, UNESCO established the International Bioethics Committee (IBC) in 1994, as the sole international body of the United Nations system in the field of bioethics. UNESCO in 1997 issued the "Universal Declaration on the Human Genome and Human Rights"[32] endorsed by the UN General Assembly on December 9, 1998. At its 32nd session in October 2003, the General Conference considered that it was "opportune and desirable to set universal standards in the field of bioethics with due regard for human dignity and human rights and freedoms, in the spirit of cultural pluralism inherent in bioethics." During subsequent years, it brought out an "International Declaration on Human Genetic Data" (October, 2003)[33] and "Universal Declaration on Bioethics and Human Rights" (2005).[34] It is important to note that in the Declaration adopted in 2005, respect for human vulnerability is promoted as one of the fundamental ethical principles for global bioethics. Although the focus of the Declaration is wider than health research, the principle of vulnerability is applicable to health care, research, and the application of technologies. This is not only applied to individuals but also to families, groups, communities, and populations since, according to the Declaration, it applies to all human beings without distinction as to who should benefit from the same high ethical standards in medicine and life science research.

Others

- Safeguarding the rights and welfare of individuals participating as research subjects in developing countries, the Joint United Nations Programme on HIV/AIDS (*UNAIDS*) embarked on a process of international consultation in September, 1997. Its purpose was to further define the important ethical issues and to formulate guidance that might facilitate the ethical design and conduct of international HIV vaccine trials and brought out a consultative document on *AIDS vaccine research 2000*.[35] UNAIDS and WHO have recently released a new version of the guidance document "Ethical Considerations in HIV Prevention Trials" (UNAIDS, 2021).[36]
- The HIV Prevention Trials Network (*HPTN*) is a global collaborative network that conducts clinical and behavioral studies on non-vaccine interventions to reduce the transmission of HIV. In 2003, the *HPTN*

developed "Ethics Guidance for HIV Prevention Research" to enhance the responsible conduct of its research activities and as a distinctive contribution to global research ethics. This was revised in 2009 and updated in 2020.[37]

- The National Bioethics Advisory Commission (*NBAC*) in USA was established by an executive order in 1995 to advise the National Science and Technology Council and other government entities on bioethical issues arising from research on human biology and human behavior. During the commission's 5-year tenure, it submitted six major reports to the White House that contained 120 recommendations on several complex bioethical issues, including the cloning of human beings, research involving persons with mental disorders that may affect decision-making capacity, research with human biological materials, embryonic stem cell research, US-sponsored clinical trials in developing countries, and protection of human research participants. Although no legislation has been passed based on NBAC's recommendations, agencies responsible for a major portion of federally funded research involving human participants, particularly the National Institutes of Health, have adopted several of NBAC's recommendations and issued research guidelines based on those recommendations.[38] President Obama's Presidential Commission for the Study of Bioethical Issues, set up to examine the US Public Health Service studies conducted in Guatemala in the 1940s, came out with a candid report in December, 2011 and recommended that research participants be protected in domestic as well as international research.[39] It also published 10 reports on ethical issues during its tenure of 8 years along with several other publications to promote bioethics education.

- In 2018, the TRUST Consortium comprising 13 partners led by University of Central Lancashire, UNESCO, INSERM, COHRED, PHFDA, University of Witwatersrand, Forum for Ethics Review Committees in India (FERCI), etc., funded by the European Commission (EC), brought out the Global Code of Conduct for Research in resource-poor settings for international collaborative research with the basic values of Fairness, Respect, Care, and Honesty while conducting research in resource-poor countries. This code is now adopted by the EC for compliance by all researchers receiving funding from them for collaborative research projects[40] and is used by more than 40 countries now. It is translated into most of the languages of these countries, including Hindi.

All the existing documents provide a largely consistent ethical framework that is still evolving in detail, especially concerning international research and research that involves vulnerable population. More important for these guidelines is the mechanism for their interpretation, application, and enforcement, which is still an outstanding challenge in the area of research ethics. Most of the guidelines remain as guidance documents without any legal status.

The Indian Scenario

National Ethical Guidelines for Biomedical and Health Research Involving Human Participants

To address the emerging new issues and reporting of some unethical studies, it became necessary for the Indian Council of Medical Research to update the 1980 guidelines and set up the Justice Venkatachaliah Committee in 1996. The revised ethical guidelines entitled Ethical Guidelines for Biomedical Research on Human Subjects were released in 2000 after extensive consultation and public debates. The revised guideline elaborated on 12 general principles stemming out of the four basic principles stated earlier and details on five specific areas, namely, clinical trials, epidemiological research, human genetics research, organ transplantation, and assisted reproductive technologies.[41] All institutions conducting medical research were required to follow these guidelines in letter and spirit and the research proposals were to be approved by a duly constituted Ethics Committee. The roles and responsibilities of the Ethics Committees and the details of the ethics review procedures were also elaborated in the chapter on "Ethics Review Procedures." In the late 1990s and early 21st century, bioethics occupied the central spot in scientific discussions due to growing international collaboration and emerging new technologies. Hence, these guidelines needed further updating, which was accomplished in 2006 as Ethical Guidelines for Biomedical Research on Human Participants with additional content on clinical trials, different types of ethical review procedures including disaster situations, the nuances of stem cell research and therapy, and the global issues related to biobanking. The assisted reproductive technologies were also updated as the related Bill was being prepared at that time. A major change was to replace the term "Human Subjects" with "Human Participants" since the latter sounded more ethical as it puts the research participants on an equal status with the researchers. Research cannot be conducted unless there are research participants and they constitute the central role in a research enterprise, whether it is human beings in person, their biological materials, or their biological data. Referring to them as "subjects" puts them in a lower pedestal, and this was considered unethical resulting in the change of the term from subject to participant.[42] Efforts were initiated to legislate these guidelines to make the provisions mandatory for all so that ethics committees exist in all institutions and quality ethical review is undertaken. Further, those violating the same can be subjected to penal provisions. However, the amended Schedule Y of Drugs and Cosmetics Act, 2005, and the Indian Medical Council (Professional conduct, Etiquette and Ethics) Regulations, 2002, from the Medical Council of India[43] already included the compliance to ICMR National Ethical Guidelines as a mandatory requirement for clinical trials and research by physicians, respectively, thus giving the most needed legal backup to the guidelines. The latest version of the National Guidelines for Biomedical and Health Research Involving Human Participants, 2017,[44] has provided a more detailed guidance related to the existing topics in view of the emerging ethical concerns and added a number of newer areas in which guidance was lacking, totaling to 12 sections. The scope of the guidelines has been expanded to include responsible conduct of research (RCR), public health research, socio-behavioral research related to health, and ethics related to biobanking in research involving biological material and datasets. The topics in earlier versions of the guidelines pertaining to informed consent, vulnerability, biological materials, and biobanking and research during humanitarian emergencies and disaster got expanded into separate sections. The first six sections are more generic, applying to all types of biomedical and health research, such as general principles, general issues, RCR, ethical review procedures, informed consent process, and vulnerability while the next six sections are more subject specific such as clinical trials, public health research, social and behavioral research, human genetics research, biological materials/biobanking/datasets, and research during humanitarian emergencies/disasters. The clinical trials section has been expanded considerably and guidance has been included regarding investigator-initiated trials, academic research, student research, multicentric trials, those involving communities, traditional systems of medicine or using new technologies, etc. The importance of a priori arrangements for post-trial access and benefit sharing after completion of research has been mentioned in several sections, and this is to ensure that the meaningful outcomes are translated into benefits for the participants or communities and do not remain limited to publication alone. The epidemiology chapter of the earlier guidelines has been replaced with the public health research section. This section has also provided specific guidance for the conduct and review of surveys, implementation research, demonstration projects, community trials, surveillance studies, program evaluation studies, etc. A new section on ethical aspects of social and behavioral research related to health has been included for the first time. In view of the sensitive nature of most of the social and behavioral research, types of deception that can be used while administering informed consent followed by debriefing of aggregate data find an important mention in the new section on ethical aspects of social and behavioral research related to health. There was lack of clarity about the requirements such as review by EC, informed consent process, and assessment of risk–benefits in research involving sensitive studies, which is addressed in this section. The guidelines discuss the need for community engagement whenever possible and to understand the requirements and health needs of the participants. In the area of genetic research and newer technologies, especially the recent CRISPR technology and the ethical dilemmas that it poses are discussed and there is a hope that this would show a way forward for research despite the challenges to human health and safety. In the Biobanking section on Biological Materials, Biobanking and Datasets, the different options for consent, maintenance of confidentiality, use of leftover clinical/research samples, transfer of biospecimens, long-term storage, return of results, and benefit sharing are explained for consideration by researchers, biobanks, forensic laboratories, and ECs. In the section on Humanitarian Emergencies and Disasters, the requirements for emergency review by the EC, prior preparedness, consent documentation, sensitivity involved in dealing with the affected community, and planning as well as protection from invasion of privacy are described, while balancing these with the need for conducting research.

Subsequently, a handbook was also prepared in 2018 and released in 2019, which gives in a nutshell the salient features of the 2017 guidelines as a ready reference.[45]

New Drugs and Clinical Trials Rules, 2019

The amended drugs and cosmetics rules, New Drug and Clinical Trials (NDCT) Rules, released on March 19, 2019, make it mandatory for all ethics committees doing biomedical and behavioral research to follow the ICMR National Ethical Guidelines, 2017 and get registered under the Department of Health Research (DHR) in addition to institutions conducting regulatory trials getting registered under CDSCO.[46] Hence, while clinical trials for marketing approval are regulated under the Drugs and Cosmetics Act and Rules, all biomedical and health research must follow the ICMR National Ethical Guidelines. In this regard, an authority has already been set up on September 12, 2019, by the DHR for registration of ECs for biomedical and health research involving human participants and a National Ethics Committee Registry created for Biomedical and Health Research (NECRBHR) to facilitate receipt and processing of applications seeking registration and to assist the authority in the discharge of its duties. A portal with the domain name "naitik.gov.in" has also been developed to facilitate registration[47] which became mandatory from September 19, 2019, onward. There is a need to harmonize the different guidelines and regulations/rules for equitable protection, whether research participants get enrolled in clinical trials or basic or applied biomedical or health or sociobehavioral research. This is a welcome development which has given teeth to the ethics guidelines to ensure compliance by all stakeholders.

National Guidelines for Ethics Committees Reviewing Biomedical and Health Research During COVID-19 Pandemic, 2020

The year 2020 ushered in a new era of global pandemic of a viral pneumonia caused by a newly discovered corona virus, SARS-CoV-2. This pandemic has brought unprecedented, major challenges for the rapid and robust ethical review of biomedical and health research including the ethical conduct of research related to COVID-19. The first human case of COVID-19, the disease caused by a novel zoonotic corona virus, was first reported in Wuhan, China, in December 2019 and the WHO declared this as a Public Health Emergency of International Concern (PHEIC) on March 11 and declared it a pandemic as it had spread to 113 countries.

There was an urgent need for comprehensive research as well as expeditious review at the shortest possible time by the ethics committees in these times of crisis while simultaneously protecting researchers and research participants. The ethics committees were encouraged to come out with therapeutic options to tackle the problem and approve studies rapidly, without compromising scientific integrity and safety of the research participants. To guide the EC members and the researchers, ICMR came out with the National Guidelines for Ethics Committees Reviewing Biomedical and Health Research during COVID-19 Pandemic in April, 2020,[48] one of the first in the world. Fast-track evaluation of research proposals, holding virtual meetings, alternate methods of obtaining informed consent, reaching out to communities and participants, and expanding the scope of vulnerable groups, to include researchers and healthcare workers are some of the highlights of this document. The guidelines also included a standard operating procedure (SOP) to facilitate emergency review of research by ethics committees. This is the best example of the dynamic nature of these guidelines which evolve depending on the prevalent ethical challenges faced by the scientific community.

BIOETHICS EDUCATION AND TRAINING

The idea of justice and fairness in human relationships and respect for life in all its forms make the subject of bioethics important in education and research. Teaching of bioethics has become an integral part of medical and life sciences curriculum in many developed countries since the early 1980s. Standards and ideals internal to the professions of medicine, dental, nursing, and allied sciences should be inculcated in the students of these professions to enable them to act in accordance with the worthy goals and expectations of healthcare institutions. Though individuals can act in accordance with principles and rules as well as their ideals to protect the rights and obligations of patients and research participants, it is essential to demonstrate these with examples and case studies applicable to different areas so that the students are able to appreciate the significance of these principles. Hence, efforts are on to introduce teaching of medical ethics in the curricula of medical and life sciences. A decade ago, the Medical Council of India (MCI) under the Graduate Medical Education (GMR), 2012 program had proposed new teaching/learning methods including a structured longitudinal program on attitude, communication and ethics through an ATCOM (Attitude and Communication) module.[49] This was to create an "Indian Medical Graduate" (IMG) possessing requisite knowledge, skills, attitudes, values, and responsiveness to function appropriately and effectively as a physician. This has been further modified in the revised GMR, 2017, as the AETCOM (Attitude, Ethics, and Communication) Module[50] for implementation in all undergraduate medical courses. It is expected that the existing network of MCI Nodal and Regional Centers and Medical Education Units of all medical colleges will be the torchbearers of this transformational change. Many short-term and long-term training programs in bioethics/research ethics were conducted by many national and international institutions/agencies including ICMR, and now Diploma and Masters courses are available in some of the institutions for those interested in the topic. Any medical practitioner/researcher who has undergone such training will be an asset to the efforts of all stakeholders to protect the dignity, rights, and welfare of the members of the society including the research participants.

CONCLUSION

Bioethics has emerged as a new discipline in the last four to five decades and is gradually growing into a multidisciplinary specialty. Though it has been a part of medical jurisprudence till now, the advances in medical sciences and their ramifications resulted in this subject becoming a specialization by itself and a new breed of trained bioethicists has come up recently to discuss and guide the healthcare institutions in ethical conduct of their activities. Law, philosophy, and social sciences are closely linked with medical decision-making, research with human participants, and the care of the terminally ill patients. Hospital ethics committees and institutional research ethics committees function as conscience keepers of the society. Bioethical discussions and debates inform individuals and the society about the new innovations and the differing values about human life so that appropriate decisions can be taken. Public policies and appropriate curriculum are the needs of the time to enable professionals to carry on with their roles and responsibilities entrusted by the public. Nevertheless, for those involved in biomedical research who are responsible for the well-being of the research participants including the students of research ethics, it has become necessary to get familiarized with the existing codes and guidelines, get appropriate training, and keep themselves updated on the newer developments and debates on the emerging issues.

REFERENCES

1. Kavirathna, Avinash C, Sharma P. Caraka Samhita, Vol. 2. New Delhi: Sri Satguru Publications; 1913. pp. 553-8.
2. Hippocrates, Jones WHS. Aphorisms I in W.H.S. Jones (trans). Hippocrates with an English translation, Cambridge, MA: Harvard University Press; 1959.
3. Hobbes T, Shapiro I. Leviathan: Or the Matter, Forme and Power of a Common-Wealth Ecclesiasticall and Civil. New Haven, CT: Yale University Press; 2010.
4. Percival T. Medical ethics; or, a code of institutes and precepts, adapted to the professional conduct of physicians and surgeons. Manchester: Printed by S. Russell for J. Johnson and R. Bickerstaff; 1803. pp. 165-6.
5. McCullough LB (Ed). John Gregory's Writings on Medical Ethics and Philosophy of Medicine, Vol. 57. Chapter [2]. Whether the Art of Medicine as it has been Usually Practiced has Contributed to the Advancement of Mankind. Dordrecht: Kluwer Academic Publishers; 1998. pp. 59-66.
6. Baker R. The American medical ethics revolution. In: Baker R, Caplan A, Emanuel L, Latham S. The American Medical Ethics Revolution: How the AMA's Code of Ethics Transformed Physicians' Relationships to Patients, Professionals, and Society. Baltimore, MD: The Johns Hopkins University Press; 1999. pp. 17-25.
7. Sass HM. Fritz Jahr's 1927 concept of bioethics. Kennedy Inst Ethics J. 2007;17(4):279-95.
8. Potter VR. Bioethics: bridge to the future. Englewood Cliffs, NJ: Prentice-Hall; 1971.
9. Reich WT. Encyclopedia of bioethics. New York: Macmillan; 1995.
10. Celsus AC. In: Greive JA (Ed). Cornelius Celsus of Medicine in Eight Books. London: Printed for D. Wilson and T. Durham; 1756. [online] Available from: https://archive.org/details/acorneliuscelsus00cels.
11. Bernard C. An introduction to the study of experimental medicine. Greene HC, trans. Medical Heritage Library, USA. Schuman; 1865. [online] Available from: https://ia902304.us.archive.org/17/items/b21270557/b21270557.pdf. [Last accessed September, 2021].
12. The Nuremberg Code, 1947. In: Trials of War Criminals Before the Nuremberg Military Tribunals Under Control Council Law No. 10, Vol. 2. Washington, DC: US Government Printing Office; 1949. pp. 181-2. Available from: https://www.loc.gov/rr/frd/Military_Law/pdf/NT_war-criminals_Vol-II.pdf. [Last accessed September, 2021].
13. World Medical Association. World Medical Association Declaration of Helsinki: Ethical Principles for Medical Research Involving Human Subjects. Finland, 1964. [online] Available from: https://www.wma.net/what-we-do/medical-ethics/declaration-of-helsinki/.
14. Beecher HK. Ethics and clinical research. N Engl J Med. 1966;274(24):1354-60.
15. The National Commission for the Protection of Human Subjects of Biomedical and Behavioural Research (1979). The Belmont report: ethical principles and guidelines for the protection of human subjects of research. Washington (DC): Department of Health, Education and Welfare. [online] Available from: https://www.hhs.gov/ohrp/regulations-and-policy/belmont-report/index.html [Last accessed September, 2021].
16. Kampmeier RH. Final report on the "Tuskegee syphilis study". South Med J. 1974;67(11):1349-53.
17. Indian Council of Medical Research. Policy statement on ethical considerations involved in research on human subjects. New Delhi, 1980.
18. Beauchamp TL, Childress JF. Principles of Biomedical Ethics. New York: Oxford University Press; 1979.
19. Beauchamp TL. The 'Four Principles' Approach to Health care ethics. In: Ashcroft RE, Dawson A, Draper H, McMillan JR (Eds). Principles of Health Care Ethics, 2nd edition. Chichester: Wiley; 2007.
20. Kant I, Beck LW. Foundations of the metaphysics of morals, and what is enlightenment? Library of Liberal Arts, 113. New York: Liberal Arts Press; 1959.
21. Tandon PN. Human genome research - Emerging ethical, legal, social and economic issues. Menon MGK, Tandon PN, Agarwal SS, Sharma VP (Eds). New Delhi: Allied Publishers; 1999.
22. World Medical Association. World Medical Association Declaration of Helsinki: Ethical Principles for Medical Research Involving Human Subjects, Scotland, 2000. [online] Available from: https://www.wma.net/wp-content/uploads/2018/07/DoH-Oct2000.pdf [Last accessed September, 2021].
23. World Medical Association. WMA Declaration of Helsinki: Ethical Principles for Medical Research Involving Human Subjects. 64th WMA General Assembly, Fortaleza, Brazil, October 2013. World Med J. 2013;59(5):199-202.
24. Bankowski Z (Ed). Proposed International Guidelines for Biomedical Research Involving Human Subjects. Geneva: Council for International Organizations of Medical Sciences (CIOMS); 1982. [online] Available from: https://cioms.ch/bioethics/ [Last accessed September, 2021].
25. Bankowski Z (Ed). Council for International Organizations of Medical Sciences (CIOMS). International Ethical Guidelines for Biomedical Research Involving Human Subjects. Geneva: Council for International Organizations of Medical Sciences (CIOMS); 1993. [online] Available from: https://cioms.ch/bioethics/ [Last accessed September, 2021].
26. Council for International Organizations of Medical Sciences (CIOMS) in collaboration with the World Health Organization (WHO). International Ethical Guidelines for Biomedical Research Involving Human Subjects. Geneva: Council for International Organizations of Medical Sciences (CIOMS); 2002.
27. Council for International Organizations of Medical Sciences (CIOMS) in collaboration with the World Health Organization (WHO). International Ethical Guidelines for Health-Related Research Involving Humans. Geneva: Council for International Organizations of Medical Sciences (CIOMS); 2016.
28. International Council for Harmonisation of Technical Requirements for Pharmaceuticals for Human Use (ICH)). Tripartite Guideline for Good Clinical Practices E6 (R1). June 10, 1996.
29. International Council for Harmonisation of Technical Requirements for Pharmaceuticals for Human Use (ICH). Integrated Addendum to ICH E6(R1): Guideline for Good Clinical Practice E6(R2). November 10, 2016. [online]

29. Available from: https://database.ich.org/sites/default/files/E6_R2_Addendum.pdf [Last accessed September, 2021].
30. Nuffield Council on Bioethics (2021) [online]. Available from: https://www.nuffieldbioethics.org/ [Last accessed September, 2021].
31. Nuffield Council on Bioethics (2021). COVID-19. Publications, Type: Policy Briefing, Date: 2020. [online] Available from: https://www.nuffieldbioethics.org/publications/covid-19 [Last accessed September, 2021].
32. United Nations Educational, Scientific and Cultural Organisation (UNESCO). Universal Declaration on the Human Genome and Human Rights. International Bioethics Committee; 1997.
33. United Nations Educational, Scientific and Cultural Organisation (UNESCO). The International Declaration on Human Gene Data. Paris, 2003.
34. United Nations Educational, Scientific and Cultural Organisation (UNESCO). Universal Declaration on Bioethics and Human Rights. Paris, 2005.
35. UNAIDS. Ethical Considerations in HIV Preventive Vaccine Research. Geneva: UNAIDS; 2020. [online] Available from: https://data.unaids.org/publications/irc-pub01/jc072-ethicalcons_en.pdf.
36. UNAIDS. Ethical considerations in HIV prevention trials. Geneva: Joint United Nations Programme on HIV/AIDS and the World Health Organization; 2021. [online] Available from: https://www.unaids.org/en/resources/documents/2021/ethical-considerations-in-hiv-prevention-trials.
37. HIV Prevention Trials Network. (2020). Ethics Guidance for HIV Prevention Research. [online] Available from: https://www.hptn.org/sites/default/files/inline-files/HPTNEthicsGuidanceDocument_2.26.20.pdf [Last accessed September, 2021].
38. National Bioethics Advisory Commission (NBAC). [online]. Georgetown University, USA: NBAC Publications; 2001. [online] Available from: https://bioethicsarchive.georgetown.edu/nbac/pubs.html [Last accessed September, 2021].
39. Presidential Commission for the Study of Bioethical Issues. Moral Science: Protecting Participants in Human Subjects Research. Washington, DC: Presidential Commission for the Study of Bioethical Issues; 2011. [online] Available from: https://bioethicsarchive.georgetown.edu/pcsbi/node/558.html [Last accessed September, 2021].
40. TRUST. Global Code of Conduct for Research in Resource-Poor Settings. 2018. [online] Available from: https://www.globalcodeofconduct.org/ [Last accessed September, 2021].
41. Indian Council of Medical Research. Ethical Guidelines for Biomedical Research on Human Subjects. New Delhi: Indian Council of Medical Research; 2000.
42. Indian Council of Medical Research. Ethical Guidelines for Biomedical Research on Human Participants. New Delhi: Indian Council of Medical Research; 2006.
43. Medical Council of India. Professional Conduct, Etiquette and Ethics Regulations, 2002. New Delhi: Medical Council of India; 2002. [online] Available from: https://www.nmc.org.in/rules-regulations/code-of-medical-ethics-regulations-2002/.
44. Indian Council of Medical Research. National ethical guidelines for biomedical and health research involving human participants. New Delhi: Indian Council of Medical Research; 2017. [online] Available from: https://ethics.ncdirindia.org/asset/pdf/ICMR_National_Ethical_Guidelines.pdf [Last accessed September, 2021].
45. Indian Council of Medical Research. Handbook on National Ethical Guidelines for Biomedical and Health Research Involving Human Participants. New Delhi: Indian Council of Medical Research; 2018. [online] Available from: https://ethics.ncdirindia.org//asset/pdf/Handbook_on_ICMR_Ethical_Guidelines.pdf [Last accessed September, 2021].
46. Central Drugs Standard Control Organization. New Drugs and Clinical Trials Rules, 2019. New Delhi; CDSCO; 2019. [online] Available from (https://cdsco.gov.in/opencms/opencms/system/modules/CDSCO.WEB/elements/dow nload_file_division.jsp?num_id=NDI2MQ== [Last accessed September, 2021].
47. Department of Health Research, Ministry of Health & Family Welfare, Government of India. (2021). National Ethics Committee Registry for Biomedical and Health Research (NECRBHR), New Delhi. [online] Available from: https://naitik.gov.in/DHR/Homepage [Last accessed September, 2021].
48. Indian Council of Medical Research. National Guidelines for Ethics Committees Reviewing Biomedical & Health Research during Covid-19 Pandemic. New Delhi: Indian Council of Medical Research; 2020. [online] Available from: https://ethics.ncdirindia.org//asset/pdf/EC_Guidance_COVID19.pdf [Last accessed September, 2021].
49. Medical Council of India. Attitude and Communication (AT-COM) Competencies for the Indian Medical Graduate. New Delhi: Medical Council of India; 2015. [online] Available from: http://mcircvizag.blogspot.com/2016/01/atcom-new-mci-attitudes- communications.html.
50. Medical Council of India. Attitude, Ethics and Communication (AETCOM) Competencies for the Indian Medical Graduate. New Delhi: Medical Council of India; 2018. [online] Available from: https://www.nmc.org.in/wp-content/uploads/2020/01/AETCOM_book.pdf [Last accessed September, 2021].

CHAPTER 2

Informed Consent Process

Urmila Thatte, Yashashri Shetty, Nayan Chaudhari

ABSTRACT

The informed consent process supports the basic ethical principle of "autonomy" in human research. In any clinical study, a written informed consent has to be obtained from each research participant as per the requirements of Good Clinical Practices (GCP) Guidelines, the 2017 National Ethical Guidelines for Biomedical and Health Research involving Human Participants of the Indian Council of Medical Research (ICMR), and New Drug and Clinical Trials (NDCT) Rules, 2019, of the Central Drugs Standard Control Organization (CDSCO). Researchers, sponsors, and investigators with their institutions should engage in designing and implementing the informed consent process. Ideally, an informed consent is given voluntarily, orally or in a written format, by the potential study participant after understanding the entire study details. The informed consent document should be approved by the Ethics Committee before it is used by the researcher to get the informed consent. It is an ongoing process and requires that the participant has the capacity to comprehend it and take an independent decision. Wherever this capacity is compromised, a legally authorized/acceptable representative's consent has to be sought. An ethics committee may approve waiver of informed consent, if scientifically justified. There are different types of consent, namely specific consent, broad consent, tiered consent and e-consent. From children and adolescents (between the age of 12 and 17 years) who are legally minors, assent has to be taken after providing them age-appropriate information in addition to consent from their parents/guardians.

INTRODUCTION

Informed consent is central to clinical research and honors the principle of autonomy/respect for participants. In ancient times in India, the physician decided the treatment for the patient and did not consider the patient's willingness to accept it. However, the physician could consult the family, community, and even the king, based on the risk involved.[1,2] A brief glance into the pages of Hellenistic practice reveals that Hippocrates (whose oath is taken by all doctors today) actually advised physicians "to hide as much as possible from patients."[3] The Latin source of the word "consent" is "consentire" which means "to feel together (con- "together" and "sentire" feel)." This does not really indicate autonomy or the right to exert one's own choice. In old French, "consentir" means "agree" or "comply" and further does not reflect autonomy.[4] It was only late in the 19th and 20th centuries that Western societal changes introduced the concept of having patients as partners in their healing. **Box 1** summarizes the major/key milestones of informed consent both in clinical and in research settings and illustrates how over the centuries, doctors have changed from being hierarchically superior to the patient and "dictating" terms for the treatment to the more democratic and partnership approach advocated now when they take an oath to protect the participants' rights, safety, welfare, and autonomy.

GUIDELINES AND REGULATIONS

Indian

Charaka Samhita and *Sushruta Samhita* (10th BC to 2nd AD) describe the circumstances when the family, community, and the king's permission could be sought to initiate a treatment but the patient's consent was not taken and the patient did not exercise her/his rights to choose as the treatment was given for the well-being of the patient.[5] In such instances, the treatment could be experimental in nature. Emerging ethical issues and discourses in the 20th century influenced the Indian Council of Medical Research (ICMR) to include the topic of informed consent in its first policy statement of 1980,[6] and the first and second revised ethical guidelines of 2000 and 2006, respectively.[7,8] In the third revision of these guidelines in 2017, namely, the "National Ethical Guidelines for Biomedical and Health Research involving Human Participants",[9] an entire chapter was devoted to the topic of Informed Consent Process. The Guidelines state in the Preface, "The latest version of guidelines has addressed the newer emerging ethical issues keeping in view the different

BOX 1: Major/key milestones in the evolution of the concept of informed consent.

- *c400 BC*: The Hippocratic texts and initial set of European literature discussed truth telling in their conduct and advised physicians to "hide as much as possible from patients."
- *1260–1325*: Henri de Mondeville, a surgeon and anatomy teacher, instructed physicians to compel obedience from patients by threatening them.
- *1746–1813*: Benjamin Rush, known as the "American Hippocrates," advocated sharing information with patients but did not advocate seeking consent or respecting patient decisions that diverge from those of the physician.
- *1914*: Legal status—Schloendorff vs Society of New York Hospital. The court granted that every adult person with sound mind has a right to decide about his or her own body, and a surgeon who operates without the patient's consent commits an assault for which he or she is accountable.[10]
- *1947*: The first formal edict for taking a voluntary informed consent in research was codified in the Nuremberg Code by the American judges while passing judgment against Nazi doctors who conducted human experiments in the concentration camps.
- *1964*: The Declaration of Helsinki emphasized on freely giving consent after the patient is explained completely.[11] The document has been revised seven times, the last being in 2013.
- *1979*: The concept of autonomy and respect for the research participant was introduced in the Belmont report.
- *1996*: The International Council for Harmonisation of Technical Requirements for Pharmaceuticals for Human Use—Guideline for Good Clinical Practice (ICH-GCP E6) R1 gives us that informed consent form is documented as a written, signed, and dated form[5] and Addendum R2 in 2016.
- *2017*: The Hippocratic Oath (now called the Hippocratic Pledge) has been modified to add the clause, "I will respect the autonomy and dignity of my patient." In addition, the clauses related to patients' rights have been shifted to the beginning of the document.[11]

privileges of individuals and communities required to live a life of dignity of our country". In keeping with this approach, the guideline describes informed consent as "*a continuous process involving three main components – offering pertinent information to potential participants, confirming competence of the individual, ensuring the comprehension of the participants and assuring voluntariness of participatio*n."

The topic of informed consent has also been covered in the sections on Responsible Conduct of Research, Ethical Review Procedures, Vulnerability, Public Health Research, Social and Behavioral Sciences Research for Health, Biological Materials/ Biobanking/Datasets, Genetic Research, and Research during Humanitarian Emergencies and Disasters. The revised ICMR National Ethical Guidelines, 2017, which are freely available online, will serve as a guide to encounter the challenges and worries raised by evolving ethical issues. Clinical researchers must, therefore, refer to these guidelines while designing informed consent documents (ICDs) and administering consent while conducting research in India. Indian GCP guidelines published in 2001[12] (presently under revision) describes 12 principles adopted from the ICMR Ethical Guidelines for Biomedical Research on Human Subjects, 2000,[7] that guide clinical research and the second principle is the "principles of voluntariness, informed consent and community agreement" that governs the informed consent process. Box 5.1 in the ICMR National Ethical Guidelines, 2017, gives the key elements to be included in the ICD.[9] The regulation that governs clinical trials in India—New Drugs and Clinical Trial Rules (NDCT), 2019[13]—which has superseded all the earlier rules, describes in Table 3, page 215, the checklist and format for an ICD. Relevant additions to this format can be made if required, e.g., option for future use of biological material(s) and return of results.

All the above guidelines specify that the sponsor develops/drafts the ICDs which are approved by the Ethics Committee (EC) and after obtaining required and essential approvals, the investigator administers the consent to the participants. In the case of an investigator-initiated study, the investigator will take up this responsibility and develop the consent documents.

International

- The Nuremberg Code, which is a 10-point statement,[14] first defined the need for voluntariness "..... *above all, participation in research must be voluntary*" and the "withdrawal" option as "*during the course of the experiment the human subject should be at liberty to bring the experiment to an end if he has reached the physical or mental state where continuation of the experiment seems to him to be impossible*".
- The Declaration of Helsinki in its first version (1964)[15] also mandated an informed consent clearly demarcating it as the responsibility of the researcher to obtain an informed consent. It describes the need for care against therapeutic misconception and suggests that "informed consent should be taken by a physician who is not involved in the investigation and who is completely independent of this official relationship." It also recommends a consent from a "legal acceptable representative as per the national legislation" in case of legal incompetence of the participant. In fact, it also recommends an "assent." Beginning in 1964, the Declaration of Helsinki has been revised several times—most recently in 2013. However, through all the versions, the basic principle of respecting the research participant remains predominant.[16]
- The revised CIOMS Ethics Guidelines of 2016 emphasize that "*This respect and concern is manifest in requirements for informed consent, ensuring that risks are minimized and are reasonable in light of the importance of the research, and other requirements discussed in this document*".[17]
- *ICH-GCP*: The International Council for Harmonisation (ICH) which is an important international reference document for clinical trials in its E6 guideline (1996)

defines informed consent as *"A process in which a subject voluntarily endorses his or her willingness to participate in a particular trial, after knowing relevant aspects of the trial".*[18]

Operationally, an informed consent is a written document that is *voluntary*, sought from *every participant* before initiating any study-related procedure and *documented* on the Ethics Committee (EC)-approved consent form that is based on currently applicable ethical guidelines and regulations and adhering to good clinical practices.

STAKEHOLDERS IN THE INFORMED CONSENT PROCESS

There are multiple stakeholders in an informed consent process. The direct stakeholders are the potential participant, legally acceptable representative, impartial witness (as applicable), the Investigator and Site, and the Sponsor while the indirect ones are the EC and Regulators who oversee this process.

For a valid and legal informed consent process, the potential participant:
- Must be given complete information about the research and his/her role as a participant and what it entails in terms of risks and benefits. This process is also referred to as disclosure of information.
- Should be competent enough to participate in the research and have the legal stature to take independent decisions and the intellectual capacity to understand/comprehend/process the information.
- Should be autonomous in the decision-making capacity and be free of undue influence, so as to voluntarily take a decision to participate or not.
- Must sign and date the ICD.

The investigator/delegated person taking consent should:
- Be appropriately qualified, GCP certified (for all types of clinical research), trained in site activities and relevant EC standard operating procedures (SOPs), and act according to them.
- If not the principal investigator (PI), a trained person should be delegated to take informed consent as per duty delegation logs. The delegated person should be able to address the queries and doubts of the participants.
- Ensure use of the latest EC-approved versions of ICDs.
- Be able to read/write/understand/communicate in the language of ICD (preferably participant's language) and have good communication skills.

The site needs to have:
- Infrastructure and space to ensure privacy and confidentiality of the participant at all phases and conduct an informed consent process as per relevant local/national regulatory guidelines/laws [especially when audiovisual (AV) recording is to be done].

The sponsor must:
- Have the resources to develop the ICD as per the protocol and applicable guidelines and laws.[9,13]
- Prepare vernacular translations and back translations as per the local site requirement.
- In case it is an academic, investigator-initiated research, this becomes the responsibility of the investigator and she/he must be trained to develop a comprehensive ICD and translate this into all the applicable vernacular languages.

COMPONENTS OF THE INFORMED CONSENT DOCUMENT

"Informed consent" has four critical requirements, namely, complete information disclosure, voluntarism, decision-making and capacity/competence (including understanding), and authorization of voluntary participation.

- *Complete information disclosure* refers to providing all relevant information to a potential participant that is essential to make an "informed decision." Information that needs to be provided to a research participant is well described in the ICMR National Ethical Guidelines, 2017, in the section on Informed Consent Process [Box 5.1 on page 50][9] and should be adhered to in addition to following the local EC SOPs.

A workshop conducted on September 7, 2018, sponsored by the Office for Human Research Protections (OHRP), Department of Health and Human Services, USA, on the topic "Meeting New Challenges in Informed Consent in Clinical Research" discussed the elements/components of an ICD that should be addressed in an ICD in order to provide complete information disclosure:[19]

- *"What is the learning behind the study? (Mention prior work that justifies the study, recognize concerns, and focus on the fact that the answer to the study question is unknown).*
- *What are the adjustments for you? (Summarize the reasons a patient might want— or not want—to participate).*
- *What will happen? Include eligibility criteria, randomization (consider metaphors), blinding, testing, treatment with alternatives, and outcome measures.*
- *Prioritize side effects to answer the questions, how bad and how often? Organize by seriousness, severity, and quantify likelihood."*

Importantly, the researcher:
- *Must give all the information she/he knows*
- *Will have relevant information based on which the potential participants decide about whether to give or refuse consent to study participation.*
- *Must provide information that would be shared with the potential participant.*[19]

- *Voluntarism* is defined as *"the capacity to make the choice freely and in the absence of coercion."*[20] Each prospective participant should read the patient information sheet and after understanding, sign the informed consent form and voluntarily agree to participate in the research.
- *Decision-making capacity* of an individual is defined as *"'the ability to understand and appreciate the benefits and risks of health decisions and to express and communicate decisions concerning health care."*[20] The decisional capacity of a research participant consists of four abilities:
  - To understand the information given
  - To appreciate the situation
  - To rationally manipulate the information
  - To communicate the choice[20]

It also depends largely on her/his cognitive abilities and voluntarism, and both cognitive impairment and compromised voluntarism can adversely affect this capacity. It is primarily the responsibility of the researcher to ensure that the potential participant has understood the purpose of research, risks, benefits associated with the research intervention, and obligations of research participation, and her/his right of withdrawing consent any time during the study. To demonstrate decision-making capacity, potential participants should be able to reasonably interpret and make a balanced decision.

Understanding the information is the crucial part of this element. The OHRP workshop, mentioned earlier, attempted to discuss ways that concepts could be explained to potential participants for them to understand better.

Interestingly, in one study, it was found that a large proportion of participants understood the informed consent form (ICF) well, but only half of them could identify atleast one risk and understood placebo and randomization.[21] Therefore, the informed consent process is very important, the manner in which the information is given to the participant so as to enhance their comprehension. This includes using the participant's language, local jargon, analogies from the local context, etc. Partnering with a local lay person in developing a contextually relevant information sheet is very useful and more meaningful.

Competency or competence is a legal notion and often confused with decisional capacity; although both describe an individual's ability to make a decision, they are different. Thus, competency is the individual's legal standing to make independent healthcare decisions. For example, a 16-year-old patient/participant may possess the capacity to decide for herself or himself but is incompetent legally.[20] In India, the participant must be above 18 years of age to be regarded as legally competent to take independent decisions.

- *Authorization*: Finally, participants must communicate their decision, given on a voluntary basis. Usually, this is in the form of signing the informed consent form with a photocopy of the signed form given to the participant.

Before administering an informed consent to the participant, all these four requirements should be ensured. An informed consent, correctly documented: (1) Provides transparency (an ethical aspiration), (2) allows control and authorization by the participant (an ethical requirement), (3) promotes concordance with participants' values (an ethical aspiration), (4) protects and promotes welfare interests (an ethical requirement), (5) promotes trust (an ethical aspiration), (6) satisfies regulatory requirements (an ethical requirement), (7) promotes integrity in research (an ethical aspiration), and (8) respects autonomy (an ethical requirement).[19,22]

In order to give a valid consent, a potential participant should understand:
- *That he or she is being asked for consent.*
- *How to exercise his or her right to give or refuse consent.*
- *What he or she is being asked to consent to (e.g., that he or she will receive an experimental medicine, which may or may not work and that blood will be collected a number of times over the research duration).*[19]

A meta-analysis,[21] which examined the extent of understanding by participants, found that almost a quarter did not understand their right to opt out of a study without giving reasons and almost half had therapeutic misconceptions and could NOT name at least one risk. Against this background, another systematic review, a good resource, examined the adequacy of informed consent for clinical trials using various tools that can be used to assess informed consent.[23]

CONSIDERATIONS IN ADMINISTRATION AND DOCUMENTATION OF CONSENT

There are certain preconditions to a written informed consent process, and these include the following:
- A written informed consent is needed from all potential participants before any study-related procedure (including physical examination, screening tests to assess eligibility, radiological tests, etc.) is performed.
- Ensure that the version of the written informed consent form given to a potential participant or her/his legally authorized /acceptable representative (LAR) that will be used is the most recent one that is approved by the EC.
- Ensure that the potential participant or her/his LAR is given the consent documents in the language she/he understands and record the same in the source document.
- Ensure that the potential participant is as comfortable as possible and while a person is being administered consent, ensure adequate privacy and time for discussion.

- If the potential participant is unable to give consent being minor or for medical reasons (e.g., psychiatric condition, dementia, and unconsciousness), the consent must be directed to the LAR using a separate informed consent form.
- In all the above situations, while ongoing of the study, if the patient/participant either for medical or for legal reason is able to give consent (e.g., a child becomes 18 years, an unconscious person regains consciousness, or a schizophrenic regains insight), then she/he should be consented directly, using a fresh consent form which should be kept in the study file with source notes explaining why she/he has been now consented. Further, her/his wish to continue in the study or not must be respected.
- Who can be a LAR? As per the ICMR National Ethical Guidelines, 2017,[9] a LAR is *"A person who will give consent on behalf of a prospective participant who, for either legal or medical reasons, is unable to give consent herself/himself to participate in research or to undergo a diagnostic, therapeutic or preventive procedure as per research protocol, duly approved by the EC"*. The participant's judicially appointed guardian (adult son/daughter for a demented father or father and/or mother for a child), if any, gets priority over others (caretakers/guardians).
- Where appropriate, the pediatric potential participant should additionally assent to enroll in the study (Refer to Section on Assent provided below) using the most recent EC-approved version.
- In case the potential participant/LAR is illiterate, then ensure that an impartial witness is present to witness the process and provide her/his signature for the same.
  Note:
  - The impartial witness must be literate and be able to read and understand the language, which the potential participant/LAR best understands and is being consented in.
  - Patients (with a different disease from the disease of the current study) or their relatives can be an impartial witness.
  - *Do not* take departmental members or ward staff or even relatives of the potential participant as an impartial witness.
  - Avoid taking the *same* impartial witness for *all* illiterate potential participants.
  - Social worker from other hospitals can be an impartial witness.
  - The witness should not be consenting the participant but should only witness the process as conducted by the qualified, delegated person.
  - Witness details must be captured on the consent form so that she/he may be contacted, if needed, by regulatory authorities.
- Discuss all the elements of the ICD with the potential participant or the LAR thoroughly. Provide a complete description of the study using nontechnical language.
- Allow the potential participant or her/his LAR sufficient time to read and understand the document and make enquiries.
  (*Note*: The potential participants or their LAR may take the ICD home to contemplate their participation.)
- The ICD consists of two parts. The first part is a Participant Information Sheet, which contains all the relevant information including the contact numbers of researcher. The second part is the Consent Form, which basically is a statement by the participant that he/she has been given all information related to his/her participation and that he/she is voluntarily consenting to participate. In studies where there is a significant risk, the consent form should also explicitly state the important components that the participant has understood. The first part should be given to the participant. The second part is to be retained by the researcher as a proof of having obtained the consent.
- Encourage inputs from family members, family physician, and other care providers, if appropriate, and, *only if* the potential participant consents to the involvement of the family in the consent process.
  (*Note:* This is very important, for example, in studies related to sensitive topics such as HIV.)
- Ensure that there is no undue influence (coercion) on an individual to participate or to continue to contribute in a trial.
  (*Note*: This is particularly important in case of including students/prisoners/institutionalized individuals in the study. Utmost care should be taken to ensure that they can exercise their right to refuse/opt out of the study.)
- Once the potential participant/LAR has agreed, the consent must be documented. Ensure that the potential participant writes her/his name, signs, and dates the document herself/himself along with the time after all elements have been discussed, all questions have been addressed, and the potential participant verbally consents to participate. The investigator *MUST NOT* write the name of the participant.
- The ICD must be signed by the participant in the presence of qualified research team members who have discussed the study with her/him and conducted the consent process.
- In case the potential participant or, where applicable, the LAR is illiterate, the left thumbprint should be taken instead of a signature. In this situation, the entire consent

process as well as documentation of the consent must be performed in the presence of an impartial witness who must be literate.
(*Note*: The thumbprint of the potential participant has to be dated and endorsed by the witness, and NOT the investigator.)

- The PI/designated member of the research team who obtained informed consent from the potential participant should also sign and date the ICD in the appropriate place after the potential participant and/or LAR and, where applicable, the impartial witness have signed. In some institutions, the witness signs after the PI/designated member has signed.
- Provide a replicate of the fully signed and dated ICD to the potential participant/LAR as the case may be. Document that this has been provided in the source notes with signature/left thumb impression of the potential participant/LAR (if applicable), impartial witness (if applicable), and the investigator.
- Retain the original ICD in the potential participant file at the site.
- The entire process, date, and time of the informed consent should be recorded in clear legible handwriting in the potential participant's source document. The time taken for administering the consent, the questions the potential participant asked, and the answers that were given should also be clearly documented.
- If the potential participant refuses consent, then this must be noted in the source documents, along with the reasons if given (this is because the potential participant can refuse participation without giving reasons).
- If there are any changes/amendments in the older version of ICD, a new version has to be approved by the EC and once it is approved, all the copies of the older version should be shredded and discarded by the study coordinator except for the copy which is placed in the master file with a stamp as "superseded." The superseded copy should be signed off by the PI. The participant should be reconsented as per EC instruction if any changes are made in the ICD during the study.
- Informed consent narrative should be written in the potential participant's source document by the member of the research team who obtained the informed consent.

TYPES OF CONSENT (WRITTEN, ORAL, AUDIO, AV, ELECTRONIC, RECONSENT, TIERED CONSENT, BROAD, SPECIFIC, IMPLIED, ETC.)

- It is generally the best practice to take a written informed consent at all times.
- A verbal consent may be recorded only in an exceptional situation with justification and after approval from EC. The CIOMS Guidelines, 2016, recommend that *when consent has been obtained orally, researchers "should provide to the ethics committee records of consent process, certified either by the person obtaining consent or by a witness at the time consent is obtained"*.[17]
- AV consenting is one way of documenting the consent process. The CDSCO, the regulatory agency responsible for clinical research in India, issued an administrative order on November 19, 2013, later amended in (2015) mandating the AV recording of the informed consent process only in case of vulnerable participants in clinical research of "New Chemical Entity or New Molecular Entity" and audio recording of the consent process in case of clinical trials of anti-HIV and antileprosy drugs.[13,24] The notification stipulated that *"AV recording of the informed consent process of each participant should also include procedure for providing information to the participant and checking for his/her understanding on such consent along with maintaining confidentiality. It should be followed with written informed consent documentation."* AV recording should be done of assent as well as of consent, wherever applicable.
- AV consenting has been shown to enhance understanding of the research process possibly because of the increased time spent by the researchers with the potential participants.[25] Although several practical challenges have been described which can be relatively easily addressed, there are a couple of ethical issues that need consideration.[26,27]
  - The participants who consent to video recording only may participate in a regulatory clinical trial as per the regulatory orders. This can clearly go against the basic ethical principle of justice. In a country such as India, it is very possible that for religious, cultural, or social reasons people may have an inherent reluctance to be recorded on video, in spite of having understood the study elements. They would like to be part of the study but will not do so because they do not want it to be video recorded.
  - The second ethical unresolved issue with AV recording is that of confidentiality: There are no clear-cut recommendations about the control a participant has over the process. There is no advice about who can review the video, whether the investigator team, EC members, and institutional and regulatory authorities, and whether the participant has the right to reject viewing of the video by any of these authorities and at what time during or after the study.
    - A study in a sample of 150 participants has shown that patients are worried about the disclosure of video recording, particularly when they have cancer or stigmatizing diseases. This is especially

true in women and younger persons, who said that they would not participate in a study because of the recording.[25]

- ◆ On July 31, 2015, the CDSCO amended the rule mandating AV recording only for studies with new chemical entities and vulnerable populations[24] and allowing only audio recording for trials related to HIV drugs and leprosy drugs. This has eased the process of informed consent; however, the benefits of AV recording cannot be denied and should be encouraged wherever possible without making it mandatory.
- ◆ Additionally, the AV recording is never monitored by the sponsor due to the confidentiality issue. The EC should regularly monitor these AV recordings to ensure that the process is being adhered to. AV recording should have an SOP. All the recordings should be archived in a retrievable manner. They should be made available to the EC or regulatory agencies for monitoring purposes or for resolving disputes.

- Of late, electronic consents have been used to document consent process. It has become a more relevant and safer method now due to restrictions created by COVID-19 outbreak. Electronic informed consent (eIC) refers to the use of electronic systems and processes that may employ multiple electronic media (e.g., text) to convey information related to the study and to obtain and document informed consent. These must also include all the essentials of informed consent in the language understood best by the participant. The interactive interface has facilitated the subject's ability to retain and comprehend the information during the consenting. It can inform any amendments affecting their continuation in the study. The participants should have the choice to use paper-based or electronic informed consent methods completely or partially throughout the informed consent process. The procedure for eIC may include an electronic method of taking the signature of the participant or the participant's LAR. In addition to an electronic record, a hard copy of the informed consent is best kept for archival and future monitoring if applicable.[28]
- *Reconsent*: This provision is always made in situations where the patient regains his/her consciousness, if he was unconscious before and therefore was not in a state of giving consent. He/she would be recruited after taking the LAR consent. If the study continues for a long time (10 years), reconsenting is advised for the participant to take a decision of continuing in the study. If a pediatric participant later becomes an adult during the trial period, reconsenting may be required.
- *Tiered consent*: The consent includes an opt-in option for future use of specimens or permission for using only some aspects of research and benefit sharing with the participants.
- *Broad/specific consent*: It allows/permits for present and future access and use of samples or data for research. There is no need to approach the participant again, if the researcher wants to do research on his/her sample in future. This is in contrast to the specific consent, wherein every time a new proposal is submitted for the use of stored samples, the donor is approached for written consent, e.g., genetic studies.
- *Implied consent*: This is acceptable for studies that provide anonymity, such as opinion surveys, but do not waive any of their rights as a research participant. The act of agreeing to fill the survey forms implies that the person concerned is ready to participate.

CONSENT FROM VULNERABLE GROUPS: ASSENT AND PARENTAL/LAR CONSENT IN CHILDREN

Assent

Assent is recommended in the ICMR National Ethical Guidelines, 2017, in addition to consent from parents/LARs for children aged between 7 and 18 years. In the same year, the ICMR has also brought out separate national ethical guidelines for biomedical research involving children with more details.[29]

Since children below the age of 18 years cannot give consent on legal grounds, this assent can be verbal/oral or written depending on the age which is supported by the parental/LAR consent, and these documents must be approved by the EC. Respecting the child's wishes is the principle underlying the assent. The child is explained the proposed research in a very simple manner, in a language comfortable to the child, and he/she understands the request to participate in the research and has a choice to accept or refuse her/his participation. If there is a discordant opinion between the child and the parent, the child's opinion will be given preference. However, if the test intervention is lifesaving and is the only option available in a trial setting, the dissent by the child may be disregarded provided parental consent and prior approval from the EC are obtained. The guidelines clearly recommend that no assent is required for children from 0 to 7 years, verbal assent in children from 7 to 12 years, and written assent for those above 12 up to 18 years. Box 6.6 of the ICMR National Ethical Guidelines, 2017, gives conditions for assent.[9]

Students' perceptions about consent and assent: A majority of students (from a study in the Middle East)[30] agreed that it was essential to take parental approval and that they would refuse to participate in research if their parents refused. Although the majority of boys felt that if it is a questionnaire-based study, then the child's approval is sufficient, whereas if variables such as blood sugar screening are planned, then both the parent and the child should agree. However, girls believed that parental consent is enough to participate in research but if adequate information is provided they felt that child's approval is enough.

It is expected that parents have an important influence on the child as shown in a study[31] that investigated parents' attitudes toward influencing their children about their participation in a specific birth cohort study. This study found that parents' attitudes toward "telling" were categorized into three communication styles depending on their insight of the risk/benefits for their children. Most parents expected that the study would benefit their children and preferred "directive telling," which was divided into "empowered telling" (provided children with a positive identity as participants) and "persuasive telling" (tried to persuade children even if they expressed disinclination). A few parents, depending on the study's potential risk, preferred "nondirective telling," which respects children's choices even if that means withdrawing from the study. This suggests that while "directive telling" may lead children to have positive associations with the study, children should be informed about the risks.

Consent Waiver

A written informed consent is mandatory for all types of clinical research, unless a consent waiver or permission for verbal consent is obtained from the EC in certain situations. People have said in surveys that they prefer to be "asked" whether they want to take part in the research even if the risk involved with participation is minimal. This is especially true in studies that use only data or are retrospective in nature.[32]

The ICMR National Ethical Guidelines, 2017[9] clearly describes the conditions where consent can be waived in Box 5.2 on page 54 and is summarized as follows:
- *When research cannot be possible without the waiver and the waiver is scientifically justified.*
- *Retrospective studies, where the participants cannot be contacted.*
- *Research on anonymized biological samples/data.*
- *Certain types of public health studies.*
- *Research on data available in the public domain.*
- *Research during humanitarian emergencies and disasters, when the participant may not be in a position to give consent.*

The guidelines go on to say that an "attempt should be made to get the participant's consent at the earliest." It is very important that the EC should make the determination about waiver of consent and not the PI. However, there is growing literature that suggests "*it may be necessary to make an exception to the general rule of informed consent for scientific research with an intervention.*"[33] The authors identified three main categories of arguments for the acceptability of a consent waiver. These include:

- *Decrease in data validity and quality*
  - Low inclusion rate leading to less accurate inclusion
  - Delay in inclusions affecting treatment outcome
  - Selection bias
  - Resentful demoralization (self-reported outcomes)
  - Hawthorne effect (self-reported outcomes)
- *Distress or confusion of participants*
  - Distress from the informed consent procedure
  - Distress from inclusion in the control arm
- *Major practical problems*
  - (Temporarily) incapacitated patients
  - Time constraints

It is important, however, to follow rules and guidelines applicable to the country of research, the SOPs of the institute, and above all the approval for waiver by EC. Additional privacy protection measures may be mandated in some circumstances.

Consent Decline

The adequacy and reasonable quality of the informed consent process can be identified using consent refusals as a metric.[34] Consent refusals and their reasons were studied from 10 studies done at one center in Mumbai over a 5-year period. The overall consent refusal rate was 21% with the rate being higher among patients in interventional studies, in pharmaceutical industry-sponsored studies, and in studies with a greater risk. Interestingly, it has been found that the consent decline rate was higher in developed countries relative to developing countries, further emphasizing the need for greater care while consenting potential participants in developing countries who may not be aware of their rights.[23]

Community Consent/Gatekeeper Permission

In epidemiological studies or socio-behavioral studies involving specific communities, their consent or gatekeeper permission is required from the head of the village/institution/agency and, if applicable, from the culturally appropriate authority and the local groups to enter the premises from where the participants would be drawn. While this is not a replacement for individual consent, which is the essential requirement of the informed consent process, giving due respect to local cultures and customs while seeking the consent/permission of the community leaders as the first step before approaching individuals is a good participatory process for meaningful public health research.[9]

INFORMED CONSENT REVIEW: ROLES OF ETHICS COMMITTEE MEMBERS

The review of the ICDs by the EC is crucial for the protection of the participant. Each EC should have its own SOP[35] to decide how to review an ICD. It is important that the nontechnical members (especially the lay member) carefully review the ICD to see if they understand any technical terms in the ICD. It is crucial that the lay person understands the ICD; so that it is comprehended easily by the participants. Additionally, it is necessary for ECs to monitor the informed consent process, which could be by reviewing signed consent forms, by observing the actual consent process, or by reviewing AV consent videos and so on. The consent process deficiencies are the most common findings in monitoring surveys done by ECs.[36]

FUTURE REQUIREMENTS

Research methods have evolved tremendously in the recent past as have materials that can be used to answer research questions. These have revolutionized the treatment of many disorders including the most recalcitrant of diseases, such as cancers. Real-world evidence studies accompanied with the use of big data in healthcare research are perhaps the most exciting advances in research methods. Advances in use of stored tissues with rapidly evolving genetic research methods pose challenges in consenting to issues related to return of results and future use of data and specimens for research. The traditional written informed consent needs to be modified in translational genomic research and evolving ecosystem of data collection. The issues of data use authorization and data privacy need to be dealt with utmost caution in line with respective global and local laws, as applicable, and development of an oversight system is definitely warranted. Social media and mobile devices are helping to recruit more participants and allowing "access" to participants remotely without the constraints of time or location. Such innovative study designs are being developed that are conducted entirely through the internet or mobile apps and have new models of online and electronic consent.[37] Throughout all this, the question that remains is how to protect the right of choice to participate or not, in the research, communicate information needed to make that choice, and design an oversight system to safeguard these core values. In the real world of the 21st century research and translational research and clinical care, the old definition of "consent" as agreement with another no longer suffices. Instead, the choice based on transparency, partnership, and shared governance is today's need.

CONCLUSION

Informed consent is the way that the autonomy of the participant is respected and is perhaps the one most important aspect of the research process. Four aspects have to be considered while obtaining informed consent- complete disclosure about the research proposal, decision-making capacity and the competence of the participant, voluntarism, and authorization (i.e., signing off on the consent). If these are respected then the informed consent process can be said to be complete.

REFERENCES

1. Shastri A. A S Sushruta Samhita Chikitsa Sthana, 6th ed, Ch. 7 47 (Ashmari Chikitsa), Verse no. 29, Part-I. Varanasi: Chaukhamba Sanskrit Samsthana; 1987. p. 42.
2. Shukla V, Tripathi R. Caraka Samhita. In: Chikitsa Sthana. Ch. 13, Verse no.176-177, Part-II. Delhi: Chaukhamba Sanskrit Pratishthan; 2007. p. 314.
3. Blacksher B, Moreno J. A history of informed consent in clinical research. In: The Oxford Textbook of Clinical Research Ethics. London: Oxford University Press; 2008. pp. 591-605.
4. Wolf SM, Clayton EW, Lawrenz F. Introduction: The past, present, and future of informed consent in research and translational medicine. J Law, Med Ethics. 2018;46(1):7-11.
5. Nandini K. Kumar. Informed consent: Past and present. Review Article. Perspect Clin Res. 2012;(3)2:18-21.
6. Indian Council of Medical Research. Policy Statement on Ethical Considerations involved in Research on Human Subjects. New Delhi: Indian Council of Medical Research; 1980.
7. Indian Council of Medical Research. Ethical Guidelines for Biomedical Research on Human Subjects. New Delhi: Indian Council of Medical Research; 2000.
8. Indian Council of Medical Research. Ethical Guidelines for Biomedical Research on Human Participants. New Delhi: Indian Council of Medical Research; 2006.
9. Indian Council of Medical Research (2017). National Ethical Guidelines for biomedical and health research involving human participants. [online] Available from: https://www.icmr.nic.in/sites/default/files/guidelines/ICMR_Ethical_Guidelines_2017.pdf [Last accessed September, 2021].
10. Osman H. History and development of the doctrine of informed consent. Int Electron J Health Educ. 2001;4:41-7.
11. Parsa-Parsi RW. The Revised Declaration of Geneva: A modern-day physician's pledge. JAMA. 2017;318(20):1971-2.
12. Central Drugs Standard and Control Organisation (2001). Good clinical practices. [online] Available from: https://rgcb.res.in/documents/Good-Clinical-Practice-Guideline.pdf [Last accessed September, 2021].
13. Central Drugs Standard and Control Organisation (2019). New drugs and clinical trial rules. [online] Available from: https://cdsco.gov.in/opencms/opencms/system/modules/CDSCO.WEB/elements/download_file_division.jsp?num_id=NDI2MQ== [Last accessed September, 2021].
14. Nuremberg Code. Trials of war criminals before the Nuremberg military tribunals under control council law, no.10, vol. 2. Washington, DC: U.S. Government Printing Office; 1949. pp. 181-182. [online]. Available from: https://history.nih.gov/display/history/Nuremberg+Code [Last accessed September, 2021].
15. Declaration of Helsinki (1964). Recommendations guiding doctors in clinical research. [online] Available from: https://www.wma.net/wp-content/uploads/2018/07/DoH-Jun1964.pdf
16. WMA Declaration of Helsinki (2013). Ethical principles for medical research involving human subjects. Available from: https://www.wma.net/policies-post/wma-declaration-of-helsinki-ethical-principles-for-medical-research-involving-human-subjects/ [Last accessed September, 2021].

17. Council for International Organizations of Medical Sciences (CIOMS); 2016. International Ethical Guidelines for health-related research involving humans. [online] Available from: https://cioms.ch/publications/product/international-ethical-guidelines-for-health-related-research-involving-humans/ [Last accessed September, 2021].
18. International Council for Harmonisation of Technical Requirements for Pharmaceuticals for Human Use (2016). Integrated addendum to ICH E6(R1): guideline for good clinical practice E6(R2). [online] Available from: https://database.ich.org/sites/default/files/E6_R2_Addendum.pdf [Last accessed September, 2021].
19. Office for Human Research Protections (OHRP) (2018). Meeting new challenges in informed consent in clinical research. [online] Available from: https://www.hhs.gov/ohrp/sites/default/files/meeting-new-challenges.pdf [Last accessed September, 2021].
20. Gupta U. Informed consent in clinical research: Revisiting few concepts and areas. Perspect Clin Res. 2013;4(1):26.
21. Tam NT, Huy NT, Thoa le TB, Long NP, Trang NT, Hirayama K, et al. Participants' understanding of informed consent in clinical trials over three decades: systematic review and meta-analysis. Bull World Health Organ. 2015;93(3):186-98H.
22. Beauchamp TL. The idea of a "standard view" of informed consent. Am J Bioeth. 2017;17(12):1-2.
23. Gillies K, Duthie A, Cotton S, Campbell MK. Patient reported measures of informed consent for clinical trials: A systematic review. PLoS One. 2018 27;13(6):e0199775.
24. Order O (2013). Audio-visual recording of informed consent of process. [online]. Available from: https://www.kem.edu/wp-content/uploads/2019/12/DCGI-Order-dated-2013-11-19-on-AV-recording-of-Informed-Consent.pdf [Last accessed March, 2019].
25. Figer B, Chaturvedi M, Thaker S, Gogtay N, Thatte U. A comparative study of the informed consent process with or without audiovisual recording. Natl Med J India. 2017;30(5):262.
26. Shetty PA, Maurya MR, Figer BH, Thatte UM, Gogtay NJ. Audiovisual recording of the consenting process in clinical research: Experiences from a tertiary referral center. Perspect Clin Res. 2018;9(1):44-7.
27. Chauhan R, Purty A, Singh N. Consent for audio-video recording of informed consent process in rural South India. Perspect Clin Res. 2015;6(3):159.
28. Office for Human Research Protections (2016). Use of electronic informed consent questions and answers, guidance for institutional review boards, investigators, and sponsors. [online] Available from: https://www.fda.gov/media/116850/download [Last accessed September, 2021].
29. Indian Council of Medical Research. National Ethical Guidelines for Biomedical Research Involving Children. New Delhi: Indian Council of Medical Research; 2017.
30. Sheyab NA, Alomari MA, Khabour OF, Shattnawi KK. Assent and consent in pediatric and adolescent research: school children's perspectives. Adolesc Heal Med Ter. 2019;10:7-14.
31. Ri I, Suda E, Yamagata Z, Nitta H. "Telling" and assent: Parents' attitudes towards children's participation in a birth cohort study. Health Expect. 2018;21(1):358-66.
32. Botkin JR, Rothwell E, Anderson R, Stark LA, Mitchell J. Public attitudes regarding the use of electronic health information and residual clinical tissues for research. J Community Genet. 2014;5(3):205-13.
33. Rebers S, Aaronson NK, Leeuwen FE Van, Schmidt MK. Exceptions to the rule of informed consent for research with an intervention. BMC Med Ethics. 2016;17:9.
34. Thaker S, Figer B, Gogtay N, Thatte U. An audit of consent refusals in clinical research at a tertiary care center in India. J Postgrad Med. 2015;61(4):257.
35. KEM IEC (2017). Full board review of submitted protocol. [online]. Available from: https://www.kem.edu/sop-ethics-committee/ [Last accessed September, 2021].
36. Shetty YC, Marathe P, Kamat S, Thatte U. Continuing oversight through site monitoring: experiences of an institutional ethics committee in an Indian tertiary-care hospital. Indian J Med Ethics. 2012;9(1):22-6.
37. Grady C, Cummings SR, Rowbotham MC, McConnell MV, Ashley EA, Kang G. Informed consent. N Engl J Med. 2017;376(9):856-67.

CHAPTER 3

Ethics of Research Involving Children

Himanshi Chaudhary, Suvasini Sharma, Naveen Sankhyan

ABSTRACT

Biomedical research involving children is essential for developing improved diagnostics and therapeutics for children. Historically, children have not been included in clinical research. Generally, the results of clinical studies in adults have been extrapolated to children. However, there has been a significant shift in the outlook in the past decade with more and more research being conducted in children. It has been recognized as a moral imperative to systematically develop clinical research involving children so that they can have equal access to new therapeutic modalities. The term "children" encompasses a wide range of age groups from neonates to adolescents with widely differing levels of growth and development and varying requirements. Hence, there are many ethical issues that need to be addressed before conducting clinical research involving children. These include the justification of research in the context of benefits to the children, preserving the rights of children, preventing any kind of iatrogenic harm, and in addition the issues of consent from parents and guardians, in the absence of parents, and assent from the children themselves.

Furthermore, carrying out research in developing countries is associated with unique challenges, some of which might be unheard of in settings of a developed country. This chapter discusses the major ethical considerations involving children as well as the unique challenges faced by researchers in resource-limited settings.

INTRODUCTION

Medical research involving children is essential for developing improved diagnostics and therapeutics for children. Historically, children have not been included in clinical research and the results of clinical studies in adults are often extrapolated to children. There has been a myriad of obstacles and hurdles to clinical research involving children. The barriers include difficulty in the development of a safe and comfortable environment for children when it comes to a new therapeutic intervention, lack of personnel trained to work with children, and problems with administration of assent/consent and maintaining the confidentiality. There has been a significant shift in the outlook in the past decade with more and more research being conducted in children. There is an increasing realization that children are not "young adults" and the physiology, pharmacodynamics, and pharmacokinetics of therapy differ from those of adults. Some diseases that are only seen in childhood or have their beginnings in childhood may amount to significant morbidity, if not managed during the early years of life. It has been recognized as a moral imperative to systematically develop clinical research involving children so that they can have equal access to new therapeutic modalities without any significant damage. However, there are many ethical issues that need to be addressed before conducting successful research involving children. These include the justification of research in the context of benefits to the children, preserving the rights of children, preventing any kind of iatrogenic harm, and, in addition, the issues of consent and assent in the absence of parents and guardians. This chapter highlights some of the major ethical considerations in research related to children, especially in resource-poor settings.

The first description of clinical research involving children dates to the 18th century when Edward Jenner on his sojourn to develop smallpox vaccine tried vaccination with cowpox vaccine in children including his own 1-year-old son. The 8-year-old James Phipps was the first child (but the 17th case) inoculated with cowpox extract as a vaccine and he developed cowpox. When he was later injected with smallpox extract, he developed no disease and was declared successfully vaccinated against smallpox.[1] Likewise, the first human antirabies vaccine was administered in a 9-year-old boy by Louis Pasteur in 1885.[2] Both Jenner and Pasteur believed that the vaccines bore prospects of direct benefit to the recipients.

Children were frequently included in clinical trials and research studies without any law and regulations till the early 20th century. The first prohibitive directive against experiments in vulnerable populations including children was issued in 1900 by the Prussian Minister of Religious, Educational, and Medical Affairs.[3] It explicitly prohibited medical interventions for the purpose of research in children. In 1931, the German Health Council released "Regulations on New Therapy and Human Experimentation" emphasizing the requirement of consent for research.[4] The Second World War saw the horror of concentration camps where the Nazi doctors allegedly conducted murderous and torturous experiments on the inmates including children without obtaining their consent. The infamous Willowbrook Experiments raised several important ethical issues including use of vulnerable, institutionalized population, lack of proper consent process, and inclusion of children in studies that could be completed in adults. In these experiments, mentally subnormal children housed at the Willowbrook State School in Staten Island (New York) were intentionally infected with hepatitis virus to study the course of this viral infection. The study lasted for 14 years beginning in 1956 and included more than 700 children.[5]

The *Nuremberg Code*, which is a 10-point code of ethics and one of the most important documents in the history of ethics in medical research, was formulated in 1947.[6] The code required an informed voluntary consent from the participants.

The mere requirement of an informed consent prohibited research involving children. It continued to be the only code of conduct for medical research until 1964 when the *Declaration of Helsinki* was formulated by the World Medical Association.[7] It is a testimony of medical ethics and principles for human experiments as part of medical research. It has undergone multiple revisions (last being in October 2013). The Declaration highlighted that "The interests of the subject must always prevail over the interest of science and society." It binds the physician with the words, "The health of my patient will be my first consideration," and the International Code of Medical Ethics declares that "A physician shall act in the patient's best interest when providing medical care." The Declaration also addressed the protection of children in research by permitting the minors to be involved in clinical research when "permission from the responsible relative replaces that of the subject." Over the years, separate guidelines for ethical considerations in biomedical research have been formulated in different countries. These include the Belmont Report in the United States of America (USA),[8] the Medical Research Council Guidelines in the United Kingdom,[9] and the European Union Guidelines.[10] In India, a policy statement on ethical considerations involved in research on human subjects was formulated by the Indian Council of Medical Research in 1980 which covered the topic of clinical research on children.[11] There have been subsequent revisions in the guidelines and the latest one, developed in 2017, is called the *National Ethical Guidelines for Biomedical and Health Research Involving Human Participants*.[12] To address the issues of ethics pertaining to children in clinical research, the National Ethical Guidelines for Biomedical Research involving children have also been formulated by ICMR in 2017.[13]

WHY RESEARCH INVOLVING CHILDREN?

Advances in biomedical research have augmented the longevity of thousands of children around the world. They comprise a vulnerable population with anatomical, developmental, physiological, and psychological differences from adults and hence require research separately for their needs. Few reasons why research involving children is necessary are as follows:

- Some diseases are confined only to children, e.g., hyaline membrane diseases, inborn errors of metabolism, and biliary atresia. Therefore, these will need research to be carried out only in children.
- There are certain diseases that affect all ages, but the etiologies and the pathophysiology concerned are different depending on the age, e.g., seizure disorder and cancer. The treatment also differs based on the etiology. Hence, unless clinical studies are carried out in children, therapeutic uncertainties related to diseases in children will prevail.
- The pharmacodynamic and pharmacokinetic profiles of the drugs in children are different from what is seen in adults. This is primarily because of differing physiologies and immature drug metabolism pathways in children.
- The spectrum of drug toxicity also could be different depending on the age and bodyweight-based drug dosages prescribed for children.
- Palatability of drugs and the type of age-appropriate drug delivery vehicle needs to be addressed in cases of children. Certain formulations (e.g., syrup) are more convenient, safer, and palatable as against others (e.g., capsules). Hence, the relevant pharmacokinetics and bioavailability of the drugs and their dosage forms and schedules need to be studied separately in children.
- Certain adult diseases have their origin in childhood. Hence, research to study their natural history is justified specially to increase our understanding of the disease and possibilities of prevention and also that of a late-onset disease for possible interventions from early years of life.
- The different stages of growth and development in children also require the researcher to clearly identify the age group to be researched and the expected outcomes.

UNIQUE CHALLENGES IN CHILDREN

Research involving children faces a number of challenges different from what is expected from research involving adults. These involve certain practical, methodological, and regulatory concerns that need further discussion.

- *Defining and measuring outcomes and other variables*: There are no normative data for comparison that is age or weight dependent. Due to this fact, describing an appropriate outcome can be challenging in the context of research involving children. It becomes even more challenging in cases of rare disorders.
- *Administering interventions and measurements*: A particular challenge with research in children is to assess the appropriateness of the methodology of research in the context of the young age of the participants. For example, in young infants, due to the small volume of blood, only a limited amount of blood can be withdrawn for research purposes. Similarly, children cannot be expected to perform accurately in tests that require a verbal response from children (e.g., assessment of sensory functions) and tests that require abstract thinking or understanding.
- *Research in small study population*: Some diseases affecting children are uncommon and require involvement of multiple centers and necessitate long periods of participant enrollment to enroll the required number of participants. To overcome these limitations, studies concerning children require long recruitment durations, multicenter collaborations, and innovative study designs to retain participants in the trials.
- *Designing and implementing long-term studies*: Long-term follow-up is particularly needed in children to assess the long-term impact of the diseases and their treatment, which may not be apparent in short-term follow-up and therefore get missed, e.g., hearing loss following administration of gentamicin in neonatal sepsis which was identified much later and led to nonuse of gentamicin in neonates. Similarly, the long- term risk of cranial malignancies developing in children following cranial irradiation for leukemia could be assessed only on long-term follow-up studies of leukemia patients, which revealed an increased frequency of neuroendocrine abnormalities, neuropsychiatric problems, and intracranial malignancies. This led to eliminating cranial irradiation as part of therapy for childhood leukemia.[14] Many other conditions also require long-term follow-up, e.g., neurodevelopmental outcomes in children with neonatal insults needing long-term follow-up of participants and requiring preventive interventions for as long as the disease occurrence is expected. Implementing long-term studies involve a lot of logistic issues—subjects may migrate, investigators may change their affiliations and interest, etc. Long-term funding may not be available and inflation may result in insufficient funds.
- *Working with families*: Families of the participants have a big role to play in research concerning children. Most of the time, the consent for participation is obtained from the parents. Their decision-making is affected by numerous social and cultural factors as well as by other influencers in the family. These may be particularly demanding for the investigators who need to be culturally sensitive to proficiently balance cultural practices with medical principles. When research involves acutely/critically sick children, the onus of decision-making lies on parents who are under extreme psychological stress; in such cases, it becomes difficult for the investigator to negotiate with the families. We also see the parental reluctance in allowing participation of their children in research concerning sensitive issues such as child abuse, familial disharmony, and substance abuse.
- *Meeting ethical and regulatory standards for pediatric research*: In all guiding ethical principles, children have been identified as a vulnerable group participating in medical research. This is specified in ICMR National Ethical Guidelines (2017) at section no. 6.5. Regulations and institutional policies restrict certain types of research on children. Research that does not directly benefit them and involves more than minimal risk for healthy children is restricted. Phase 1 clinical trials involving healthy volunteers are not usually allowed to include children as participants. Likewise, standard of care versus new drug efficacy trials require greater scrutiny if they involve children. These add to the administrative woes of the investigators and delay the planning and implementation of research.
- *Training and retention of clinical investigators*: There is also a shortage of properly trained investigators who are trained in clinical research involving children. Most of the pediatric training programs are inclined toward clinical care rather than research. There is a need to include the requirements of pediatric research in the university curriculum.

CHALLENGES IN THE DEVELOPING WORLD

Developing countries have 85% of the world's population. However, they contribute to only 27% of the world's medical literature.[15] As per statistics, nearly half the deaths in women and children in developing countries are from preventable causes.[16] Hence, there is a need for robust scientific research that studies the local epidemiology and disease pattern, care-seeking behavior, etc. It can help guide better management of these conditions. Carrying out research in developing countries is associated with unique challenges, such as cultural practices, financial status, and healthcare facilities.

- *Informed consent process*: Informed consent forms the foundation of ethics pertaining to research. It can be problematic in the context of a developing nation where the low education level of the participant may not allow a complete understanding of the research as the consent form is most of the time in English. In such situations, it is recommended that the consent form is translated into the vernacular language with limited use of technical terms. There is a provision of waiving off the written consent and accepting verbal consent in exceptional cases, but it has to be allowed by the ethics committee (EC) provided the process is witnessed by a literate-independent individual and the same is documented.

- There are issues with autonomous decision-making. Many populations across the developing nations are family and community oriented. Permissions to participate in research are usually given by the elder members of the family or chief of community. So, the consent is not entirely voluntary in such cases. When parents are not available, identifying a legally acceptable representative who can give genuine consent is another difficult challenge.
- *Culturally unacceptable interventions*: Certain treatment and interventions may not be culturally acceptable in certain communities. These are faced with strong criticism and boycott from society, e.g., education on sexually transmitted diseases to school children may not be accepted in certain communities. Hence, research appropriate to the culture and ethnicity should be carried out to prevent any harm to the participants and prevent social divide.
- *Legal requirements*: Certain legal issues may arise in relation to confidentiality aspects. For example, immigrants may feel threatened if they provide medical/demographic information, substance abuse by children may have legal implications which might dissuade the research, and having adolescents as participants, who might possess decision-making capacity to provide assent, but would still require a parental consent as a legal requirement.
- *Therapeutic misconception*: The chances of "therapeutic misconception," i.e., the research participant confusing treatment with research, are much more likely to occur in research-constraint settings as participants with low levels of literacy are less likely to fully comprehend the issues in research being different from those of treatment.
- *Financial inducement*: The chances of financial inducement of the parents or guardians are high in resource-poor settings of developing countries which may cloud their judgement in consenting on behalf of their child's participation in research.

ISSUE OF ASSENT/CONSENT

Assent

Children are considered as "minor" and therefore lack the legal and intellectual capacity to make decisions. Hence, it lies in the prerogative of parents or a legally authorized/acceptable representative (LAR) to allow a child's participation in a study. Explaining in legal terms, a LAR is "An individual or judicial or other body authorized under applicable law to consent on behalf of a prospective participant to participate in research or to undergo a diagnostic, therapeutic, or preventive procedure as per research protocol." Researchers may involve children in discussions related to research and seek their agreement to participate as per their intellectual capacity and the ability to take decisions.

The permission obtained from the parents/LAR for the child's involvement in the research is termed "consent" and when the child agrees to participate in the research, it is termed "assent." Parental/LAR consent is required in all instances.

A child's assent should be obtained through the provision of age-appropriate information and considered as a child's affirmation to participate in the research, which should be voluntary. It should take into account the intellectual level and the child's ability to take decisions. Children can have a variable understanding of the concepts based on their reading abilities and social and cultural practices. Unlike informed consent, assent is not a legally binding process but ethically important. It is an opportunity for the children to express their feelings and viewpoints regarding their participation in the research. It is symbolic of respecting children's rights and responsibilities during the research process. It requires that the participants should have a basic understanding of their role in the research.

Lowes et al. identified that children above 7 years of age possess necessary cognitive development to be able to give consent.[17]

Legally, there is a "mature minor doctrine" in common-law rule of US, Canada, and Australia that allows an adolescent (above 14 years in US and 16 years in Canada and below 18 years in Australia) who is capable of making medical decisions to give consent for medical care without involving the parents. These instances include blood donation, emergency care, sexual and reproductive health such as pregnancy, contraception and sexually transmitted diseases, drug treatment, drug abuse, and mental health care. In all these situations, the adolescent is considered as a mature minor if the requisite intelligence, understanding, training, experience, economic independence, and marital status for making independent decisions by themselves exists. In the Indian context, the National Ethical Guidelines for Biomedical and Health Research Involving Human Participants (2017) have stated in its section on assent that "There is no need to document assent for children below 7 years of age." If the child is between 7 and 12 years of age, then verbal or oral assent must be obtained in the presence of the parents/LAR. For children aged 12–18 years, written assent is suggested. All assent forms have to be signed by the parents/LAR. Many adolescents may have the intellectual capacity and maturity to give consent like adults. However, this is not permitted by law and hence their consent is still termed assent and the consent of the parents/LAR is required. If involvement of parents/LAR will affect the validity of the study, waiver of consent can be taken from the EC, for example, in studies of sexual habits of adolescents, where parental consent may not be possible. However, if a child seven years of age refuses to cooperate with research requirements such as blood drawing, it should be taken into account by the researcher.

Informed Consent

It protects an individual's autonomy and preserves the basic human right of freedom of speech. A person, after understanding the various aspects of research being carried out, can voluntarily decide whether she/he wants her/his child/ward to be a participant of the research or not. The detailed information must be written down in a simple, easy-to-understand format and in a language that he/she can read and understand. A copy is given to the parent/LAR and to the children from whom written assent could be taken. A signed copy of the same must be kept by the investigator as well as provided to them. A thumb impression can be taken in place of signatures for those who cannot sign or are illiterate. In such an instance, there should be an impartial witness who is literate and knows the local language understood by the parent/LAR who will put her/his signature after witnessing the consent process. The participants need to be assured that their confidentiality will be maintained, and all interventions/investigations will be performed after prior assent/consent.

PROTECTION OF THE INTERESTS OF THE CHILD

The National Ethical Guidelines for Biomedical Research Involving Children, 2017, addresses issues related to the ethical recruitment of children in medical research. Certain provisions have been laid down for safeguarding the interests of child participants in clinical research:
- *Membership of Ethics Committee (EC)*: For research that involves children as participants, the EC should comprise at least one member with pediatric expertise or such a person could be invited as an expert for consultation in the interest of the participants. The expert should be independent of the researcher and sponsors.
- *Data and safety monitoring boards (DSMB)* are established in addition to EC to safeguard the interests of participant children so that any harm that can happen will be identified at the earliest and a decision can be taken on whether to continue or not with the study.
- The studies involving children should be carried out in a child-friendly environment. The investigators should have expertise in the field in which the research is being carried out. If there is less experience, then the research should be overseen by a mentor/senior researcher who has more experience in that field pertaining to children.
- Maintaining the confidentiality of records of patients is also the responsibility of investigators. It should be stated explicitly on the form that the information collected shall not be disclosed to anyone. All records must be safely kept for a period of at least 3 years after the study is completed. Documents related to regulatory clinical trials must be archived for 5 years after the completion/termination of the study or as per regulations. Data may be archived for a longer period depending on the study design and the need for longer follow-up.
- *Payments*: The payment that is offered for participation of the child must not be considered as an incentive for parents/LAR to enroll their children/ward in a study. The investigators should bear expenses of research participation. Reasonable reimbursement of the money spent in any aspect of study (travel allowance for follow-up, wage loss of parents/LAR, other incidental expenses, etc.) should be made. Medical services should be provided to the participants free of cost. Protocols and informed consent should mention clearly the details of the expenditure involved and payments to be made to the participants. If incentive payments are used for the recruitment and retention of participants in the studies, they should have the *a priori* approval of the EC. It is important that the parents stay away from any undue influence that might tempt them to enroll their children in research because there is no personal risk involved for them and there may be some financial returns. Hence, it is important to balance the incentives paid to the parents to ensure their participation and to protect the interests of the children who are participating.

RESEARCH IN SPECIAL SITUATIONS

- *Research involving neonates*: Research involving sick neonates has yielded some very important advances in neonatal care and management. Neonates are considered the most vulnerable group in the research involving children. The long-term outcomes in relation to drug safety and effects of the intervention can be assessed only after long-term follow-up. There are various problems associated with it. First, there are concerns of informed consent, which is taken from parents, most of whom may be emotionally distraught when such consent is sought. Therefore, there is usually a lack of clarity in this matter relating to enrollment. The consent is usually sought for interventions in conditions, which are often life-threatening [e.g., use of surfactant, use of extracorporeal membrane oxygenation (ECMO)] and require a quick decision to be made on the part of the parents. In these circumstances, researchers have recommended "continuous consent" wherein informed consent is reobtained at multiple occasions with the ongoing developments in the research rather than being a one-time prerecruitment process. As per recommendations, all efforts have to be made to safeguard the interests of a newborn baby.

Ethics committees dealing with research involving neonates should have at least one member with expertise in neonatal care and research and they should carefully inspect all newborn-based studies for any potential risks for the participants. There have been recommendations favoring research in older children and non-sick newborns before being conducted in sick newborns.

- *Research involving minor parents*: In the guidelines for children provided by ICMR,[13] it is stated that a minor parent cannot give consent. In situations where both parents are minors, their baby should be avoided for research enrolment. In such an instance, the consent of a legally acceptable representative is required. In contrast, in the US and Canada, minors can be granted *emancipation* for not involving parents in decision-making which may not necessarily be granted to the minors themselves. However, within the US and Canada, laws differ on the nature of involvement in research and age for minor parents. In some states, minors who are parents may be in the paradoxical position of being able to permit treatment on behalf of their child but not on their own behalf.[18]

  It is thus prudent to refrain from involving minor parents in research unless the research is specifically targeted to study and benefit this group.

- *Research in emergency settings involving children*: Certain research studies are carried out in emergency settings to determine the emergency intervention, which offers predictions of benefits to the patient. These must take place immediately even in the absence of informed consent from the parents. Such situations warrant deferred consent where the information regarding the research is divulged sequentially to the parents. They are given basic limited information at the beginning, followed by full details later. In the absence of parents, a LAR can give consent during the emergency settings. However, an advance approval from the EC should be taken for such protocols.

- *Research involving adolescents*: Adolescents differ from both adults and children in many aspects. Most guidelines recognize that adolescents have the capacity for independent decision-making and can provide consent themselves. However, they need protection and guidance for which their decisions must be supervised by the parents/LARs. Therefore, when seeking consent from the parents, it is also important to take informed assent from the participating adolescents. Certain adolescent-related research tends to address sensitive issues such as sexuality and substance abuse. Sometimes, when adolescents are intelligent enough to understand the implications of what is being proposed in the research proposal, a provision of waiving off parental consent by the EC concerned may be considered where parental permission may affect the validity of results, e.g., surveys involving the use of contraceptives/risky behavior among adolescents. Informed written assent must be obtained from the participants in such cases by using a simplified Patient information sheet (PIS) which they can comprehend and then agree to take part in the proposed research.

  During such research, the investigator also faces the dilemma of reporting this reportable behavior to appropriate authority. Therefore, first, such research should be undertaken by someone who is acquainted with the unique aspects of adolescent development. Second, confidentiality and anonymity must be maintained related to sensitive issues. Local beliefs and social stigmas must be kept in consideration while preparing such research protocols.

- *For community-based studies*, help can be sought from local youth advisory committees in exploring ethical issues and including youth in designing research. The research must be submitted and reviewed by the EC.

CONCLUSION

Scientifically designed and conducted research involving children is essential and beneficial for advancing health care of children. There are certain ethical concerns that are unique to research involving children and need to be addressed. The research requires a strong sense of responsibility preserving a balance between the scientific necessity of involving children in research and the ethical requirement of preventing any harm to the child. Research should be designed in a way that protects the welfare of these vulnerable participants. Informed consent and individual assent are of utmost importance and children should be allowed to participate in the decision-making based on their developmental status. All the stakeholders—investigators, sponsors, government agencies, law makers, EC members, parents/LAR—have a role to play in facilitating excellence in research while protecting interests and well-being of children.

REFERENCES

1. Riedel S. Edward Jenner and the history of smallpox and vaccination. Proc Bayl Univ Med Cent. 2005;18(1):21-5.
2. Rappuoli R. Inner Workings: 1885, the first rabies vaccination in humans. Proc Natl Acad Sci. 2014;111(34):12273.
3. Boss RD. Ethics for the pediatrician: pediatric research ethics: evolving principles and practices. Pediatr Rev. 2010;31(4):163-5.
4. Sass HM. Reichsrundschreiben 1931: pre-Nuremberg German regulations concerning new therapy and human experimentation. J Med Philos. 1983;8(2):99-111.

5. Goldby S. Experiments at the Willowbrook State School. Lancet. 1971 10;1(7702):749.
6. Ghooi RB. The Nuremberg Code—A critique. Perspect Clin Res. 2011;2(2):72-6.
7. World Medical Association (2018). WMA Declaration of Helsinki- Ethical principles for medical research involving human subjects, 1964 (last amended in 2013). [online] Available from: https://www.wma.net/policies-post/wma-declaration-of-helsinki-ethical-principles-for-medical-research-involving-human-subjects/ [Last accessed September, 2021].
8. Office for Human Research Protections, U.S. Department of Health & Human Services [Internet]. (2018). The Belmont Report, Office of the Secretary, Ethical Principles and Guidelines for the Protection of Human Subjects of Research, The National Commission for the Protection of Human Subjects of Biomedical and Behavioral Research, 1979. [online] Available from: https://www.hhs.gov/ohrp/regulations-and-policy/belmont- report/read-the-belmont-report/index.html [Last accessed September, 2021].
9. UKRI Medical Research Council. (2019). Policies and guidance for researchers. [online] Available from https://mrc.ukri.org/research/policies-and-guidance-for-researchers/ [Last accessed September, 2021].
10. European Commission. European Union. Ethics - Horizon 2020 Online Manual. [online] Available from: https://ec.europa.eu/research/participants/docs/h2020-funding-guide/cross-cutting-issues/ethics_en.htm [Last accessed September, 2021].
11. Sanmukhani J, Tripathi CB. Ethics in clinical research: the Indian perspective. Indian J Pharm Sci. 2011;73(2):125-30.
12. Indian Council of Medical Research. National Ethical Guidelines for Biomedical and Health Research Involving Human Participants. New Delhi: Indian Council of Medical Research; 2017. [online] Available from: https://ethics.ncdirindia.org/asset/pdf/ICMR_National_Ethical_Guidelines.pdf [Last accessed September, 2021].
13. Indian Council of Medical Research. National Ethical Guidelines for Biomedical Research Involving Children. New Delhi: Indian Council of Medical Research; 2017. [online] Available from: https://ethics.ncdirindia.org//asset/pdf/National_Ethical_Guidelines_for_BioMedical_Re search_Involving_Children.pdf. [Last accessed September, 2021].
14. Raymond-Speden E, Tripp G, Lawrence B, Holdaway D. Intellectual, neuropsychological, and academic functioning in long-term survivors of leukemia. J Pediatr Psychol. 2000;25(2):59-68.
15. Fathalla MF. Tapping the potential for health research in developing countries. Bull World Health Organ. 2004:82(10):719-810. [online] Available from: https://apps.who.int/iris/handle/10665/269255.
16. World Health Organization. Children: improving survival and well-being. Geneva: World Health Organization; 2020. [online] Available from: https://www.who.int/news-room/fact-sheets/detail/children-reducing-mortality [Last accessed September, 2021].
17. Lowes L. Pediatric nursing and research ethics: is there a conflict? J Clin Nurs. 1996;5:91-7.
18. Institute of Medicine (US) Committee on Clinical Research Involving Children; Field MJ, Behrman RE, editors. Ethical Conduct of Clinical Research Involving Children. Washington (DC): National Academies Press (US); 2004. [online] Available from: https://www.ncbi.nlm.nih.gov/books/NBK25557/.

CHAPTER 4

Ethical Issues in Epidemiological Studies

Prashant Mathur, Narendra K Arora

ABSTRACT

Epidemiological studies provide critical information on ill-health and diseases at the individual and population levels. They are used to shape up interventions, monitor them, and provide a robust evidence base. The ethical issues emerge from the interaction of the researcher (most often, the clinician) and the study participant at individual or community levels. The general principles of health research ethics are enshrined in such studies also. However, we have explained a few of them which need better explanations to practitioners of epidemiology, informed consent, protecting the welfare of research participants (including vulnerable participants), privacy and confidentiality, sociocultural contexts of research, ethics review, public trust, conflict of interest, and obligations to communities. In each of these sections, examples are provided to explain the issue. Epidemiological studies overlap with public health research, trials, operational/implementation research, and surveillance. Some key ethical issues relevant to epidemiological studies are described in this chapter.

INTRODUCTION

Epidemiology is a science of public health, which investigates how, when, and where, in the population are the health-related events occurring and distributed. Epidemiological studies also explore all the determinants of health and disease (causes, risk factors) in a specified population. A key feature of epidemiological studies is that they measure disease outcomes in both healthy and diseased or at risk population. Evidence generated from these studies describes the strength of association and not causation.[1] It supports disease surveillance, monitoring, laboratory research, and evaluation of health programs. Epidemiological information is important for addressing health problems of the community, whereas clinical research studies involve either individuals or a small group as the target population to improve clinical care. For example, clinical research on vitamin A deficiency in children improves pediatric ophthalmic practice to reduce night blindness, while the epidemiological studies on large-scale vitamin A supplementation have evolved into National Health Programs. Such efforts continue to establish it as one of the important strategies for child survival. The Framingham Heart Studies conducted for over several decades provided sound epidemiological evidence on the associated risk factors for cardiovascular diseases for planning strategies for prevention and control.[2]

Epidemiological studies usually involve a large number of participants and data sets. Some of them are carried out over long periods and are expensive. Thus, all technical, practical, and ethical components of the study require attention while planning such studies. This chapter addresses some of the major ethical issues likely to be encountered in epidemiological settings in developing countries, including India.

EPIDEMIOLOGICAL STUDY METHODS

Epidemiological studies investigate the clinical, laboratory, and behavioral aspects of health and their interactions.

Observational Studies

These studies observe and record preset parameters within defined population groups over specified periods and frequencies. The main types of study designs are as follows:

- *Cross-sectional studies*: These are carried out in a defined population. These studies include either the whole population or a random sample of the population to study the parameters of interest. The investigators come in contact with the study participants only once in a defined period. Cross-sectional studies aim to assess either different population health characteristics or test hypotheses to detect disease causative or risk factors. These studies are good for estimating the prevalence of the disease, agent, or risk factor in the population. The information is usually collected through structured questionnaires and tools.
- *Case-control studies*: These are used to compare past exposures to risk factors among those individuals who

have the disease and those who do not, and to compare them for certain characteristics such as age, sex, socioeconomic status, and geographic location. Case–control studies are done by either examining the available patient records or interacting with the study participants. In the former, informed consent may be waived off if the data is anonymized and this is determined by the Ethics Committee (EC).

- *Cohort studies*: These types of epidemiological studies are carried out on a group of individuals who are exposed to the common risk factor of interest and followed-up over a long period till the disease outcome of the study is attained. The rates of disease occurrence are measured and compared with the identified risk factors. These studies require a large number of participants for a long time and involve questionnaires, medical examinations, and sometimes laboratory investigations. Although individuals are being followed up as a group, it is essential to precisely identify every individual in that group who has to be studied. To study the influence of environmental factors on an individual's health, data from interviews, questionnaires, medical records, various registers, and biological materials from the sources of information is required. Ethical issues are to be considered at all stages of such studies.

Experimental Studies

The investigators study the effects of some interventions (drug, devices, therapy, procedure, health education, and awareness or other interventions) in the population over a while. These studies are generally randomized controlled trials (RCTs). Some of these, such as new drugs and vaccines which are clinically evaluated in the community, may come under the purview of the Central Licensing Authority (Drug Controller General of India) as per the New Drugs and Clinical Trial Rules (NDCT Rules) 2019.[3] In RCTs, the participants should be explained on the possibility of use of placebo or standard care as one of the arms of the trial as per the randomization process.

ETHICAL CONTEXTS IN EPIDEMIOLOGICAL RESEARCH

The ethical guidelines for research on human participants apply to epidemiological research as well. The basic principles of bioethics (beneficence, nonmaleficence, autonomy, and justice) are pillars of any epidemiological ethical guidelines.[4] Based upon the area of interventions, all ethical concerns and issues should be contextualized to the local socio-cultural environment. However, these contexts change over time. For example, earlier, it was not considered culturally appropriate for a woman to be interviewed by unknown men. But with time and changes in societal norms, people have started to accept these changes. To address these changing requirements and to meet future challenges, ethical issues and perceptions also adapt dynamically. Epidemiological studies are an interplay between the standard models for public health (that directs to protect public welfare) and clinical medicine (that promotes the welfare of the individual). The guidelines on ethical standards of practice should not confine the research innovation, methods, or scientific creativity. ECs should provide a framework to maintain and enhance scientific quality, rigor, and accountability.

Few important guiding principles laid out by the Council for International Organizations of Medical Sciences (CIOMS) for epidemiological research are given below:[5]

- Enhance sensitivity in ethical aspects for epidemiological studies
- Adopt ethical standards in the epidemiological study design
- Encourage meeting high professional standards and quality research with humane attitudes

Some unique issues in the ethical perspective of epidemiological studies are:

- Community beneficence versus individual autonomy
- Information disclosure
- Stigmatization or harm to an identifiable community or group
- Conflict of interest due to interaction with special interest groups
- Regulatory versus ethical issues

The ethical concerns and issues are interwoven with each other, and duplication may be observed in the sections discussed ahead.

SPECIFIC ISSUES IN EPIDEMIOLOGICAL RESEARCH

Informed Consent

Inherent ethical issues stem from the competence to provide informed consent, freedom from coercion, accuracy to translate information on potential risks and benefits, alternatives to study participation, and the liberty to cancel the informed consent and voluntary withdrawal from the study without penalty.[6]

Challenges

The conceptualization of the informed consent form is based on the western-based thinking that all adults are capable of taking independent decisions regarding their study participation.[7] Illiteracy associated with the inability of the participant to read is one of the major obstacles in developing countries and even for those who can read it, comprehension becomes an important limiting factor. The participants may have different levels of understanding of the research, dependent on the time spent in explaining it.

In traditional Indian societies, the individual's autonomy to give consent is chiefly guided by the agreement of household elders, friends, relatives, or even the community. A study undertaken in a rural area of Haryana aimed to understand the decision-making process in clinical research participation.[7] Of the 59 households interviewed, only 36.8% of the participating men and women agreed to provide complete independent consent, while the remaining sought consultation and opinion. In contrast, 98.2% were willing to participate in interview-based surveys and 86% agreed to participate in studies involving blood sample collection. From this, we can conclude that there was reluctance to be part of vaccine and drug trials due to the "risks" involved. Also, most people were not familiar with the word "research" and the meaning to "participate" in it. For some respondents, familiarity and respect for the medical fraternity overcame the fear of the risk of being involved, and they only foresaw the benefits (therapeutic misconception). Few were willing to participate in research since they felt that there was nothing to lose. Those who felt that they were "well" expressed their desire against participation. This inability to understand the implications of participation puts forth the responsibility on the investigator to explain the purpose of the study and its associated benefits and risks. The communities may perceive such studies as threatening the safety of the local participants in international collaborations. The participants must be made to understand that their participation is not compulsory and that they have the power to withdraw or refuse participation in the study without the fear of any consequences. Therefore, studies being undertaken in communities in developing countries require additional efforts of investigators to make the participants understand the full contents and implications of their participation in the study.

Enabling Methods for Obtaining Informed Consent

In many circumstances, obtaining consent over some time through consultation would be more suitable than obtaining it on the spot. Consent can be taken in stages in certain special circumstances.[8] It could begin with community-level consultations and then with the selected participants. This would provide them with more than one-time interaction with the research team and enable them to give free consent genuinely.[9] The use of demonstration tools would be useful in explaining them the project and clarifying their doubts. In social science research, a "flower diagram" was found to be useful in explaining risks and benefits during an interactive session.[10] Other ways of documenting agreement to participate should be explored, for example, audiovisual recordings. The research team must be well trained in communicating with the participants, and if needed the senior researchers must accompany the team. Some studies have shown that with prior consent, the response rates decline enough and may lead to selection biases, which would limit the generalizability of the results to the entire population.[11]

In developing countries including India with diverse cultures and dialects, the content of the consent form should be prepared in their respective local language; it needs to be simple and understandable in the cultural context.[7] As this can affect the way information is being conveyed to the research participants, especially in multicentric studies, this needs to be implemented and handled at every study site. Information routines must be adjusted/packaged to meet the demands, thus allowing research participants to easily choose their preferred level of detail. In longitudinal studies, if the participants do not take all the provided information, then this can affect their participation at later stages, wherein they may realize that their participation demanded more involvement than what they had anticipated. To avoid such situations, testing the informed consent to assess the understanding of its content by the population to be studied and its impact on participation would be useful in revising the document based on the need.

Epidemiological studies include validation of previously completed studies. Subsequent studies during interim analysis may negate the benefits demonstrated by the earlier studies. In the CARET (Carotene and Retinol Efficacy Trial) study conducted in the US, the interim analysis failed to demonstrate the beneficial effects of carotene and vitamin A administration for lung cancer prevention and thus compelled the authorities to discontinue its use based on earlier studies. In such instances, the continuation of carotene and vitamin A administration till the end of the study period to attain scientific validity would have exposed the participants to unnecessary potential risks of supplementation without any benefits.[11] This becomes an ethical issue when obtaining informed consent and explaining the risks and benefits of participation. Thus, investigators should consider that a consent form could be changed based on the emerging scientific facts for which re-consent may be required during the conduct of the study.

Electronic data exchange and internet technologies play an important role in the effective coordination of health care and research. It would entail repeated visits to the participant's data by various researchers at varying intervals. The participants can opt for specific options ("in" and "out") for seeking their participation in the review of their records.[12] However, in developing countries, such accommodations to assess the ethical implications of e-consent will be challenging, mainly due to illiteracy in electronic communications and unreliable internet connections.

Though the study may not intend to cause harm, ethical issues may arise when using sources such as occupational records, medical records, and tissue samples, as prior consent was not given. Individuals or their public representatives could be informed before beginning the study that their data could be used for further analysis and how confidentiality will be ensured at all stages.

Ethical aspects of using the power of access to personal data are considered when a third party accesses the data without participants' consent. Many times, epidemiologists are called upon by organizations and government agencies as the third party for undertaking specific analysis of previously collected data sets.[13] In such scenarios, the EC may direct obtaining consent from the concerned individuals or based on appropriate justifications, EC may allow access to de-identified data without consent. Such considerations to the breach in confidentiality of concerned study individuals, are governed on grounds like significant public benefit outweighs the risk or any harm on the individuals. Data access and sharing protocols must be in place at the institutional level. ECs must be consulted to clarify and specify such concerns and seek their approval for waiver of consent. This has been explained in the ICMR National Ethical Guidelines under the section 8.4.4 with examples.[14]

For communities in which collective decision-making is customary, the leaders chosen by the communities or culturally appropriate authority may express it as a collective will.[7] However, study participation refusals still need to be respected. The study investigators and the ethics committees must consider if the community leaders are speaking on behalf of the group in its interest (gatekeepers) and only after consulting and agreement from the members of the community. Representatives of the community or group should be encouraged to participate in designing the study and its ethical elements as a good participatory practice exercise. Investigators should be sensitive to the process of forming such community groups by following any local norms and sensitivities involved and must always respect the rights of different groups, mainly the underprivileged.

The blanket/broad consent strategy is adopted by some researchers doing occasional studies in communities, for example, post-disaster research, wherein their representatives provide blanket approval to the investigators. In such situations, a blanket requirement for consent from every participant in observational research can produce bias in the study findings. So, it is to be seen to what extent it is appropriate in ensuring autonomy and privacy to the individual study participant. In community-wide studies, the focus should be directed at avoiding possible exploitation, rather than trying to obtain individual informed consent. Openly improving community consultation processes for a better clarity may be of value, in avoiding possible paternalistic decisions made by the investigator.[15] This also facilitates building trust for obtaining individual consent as required by the ICMR guidelines.[14]

In follow-up studies where data is collected over a long time, the issue to be considered is whether one-time consent is enough or repeated consent is required.[16] The initial consent can consider the long-term agreement for participation and accessing data. Given changes that could occur in the study protocol or scientific information related to the study, the ethical requirements must be made available for reconsideration by the participants and this will require the EC's approval. Very few investigators can predict the period of a long-term follow-up study, as they are driven by uncertainties over funding, researchers' motivation levels, and the obvious impact of initial results, all of which are likely to alter the frequency of follow-ups. As previously discussed, the changes in ethical practices are common and informed consent that was obtained years ago may no longer be valid.

Many ECs have demanded to exclude patients who do not or cannot consent. It is evident from the literature that participants who consented to health surveys were more likely to be young, healthier males, nonsmokers, better educated, and from higher socioeconomic status. In an observational disease registry, consenting adults were both predictably and unpredictably different from those who did not consent.[17]

The participants, public, and professional organizations must consider the implications of blanket/broad consent from every participant.

The study investigators are obligated to disclose all the relevant information to enable patients or other individuals to take an independent decision on their participation. Potential participants in epidemiologic research must be detailed on the extent to the protection of confidentiality and the study intent as well as the potential uses of the collected data that contain personal identifying information. The ECs need to safeguard participants when deception techniques are used in research for investigating some highly sensitive issues when the participants are unaware of it. De-briefing the participants afterward should be encouraged. The investigator may disclose new information obtained during the course of the study, which the participant would consider for continuing her/his consent for participation. Steps must be taken to ensure that the study participants (including minors) clearly understand the given new information. Informed consent must be able to explain the study and any larger implications of intended research to a layperson. Despite due payment being received for their participation, the consent to participate in the planned intervention must be voluntary without coercion, or manipulation, or any undue incentives. Ethical concerns arise when the intended and potential uses of data are not well communicated to the participants. This is particularly true for data in the public domain and for which consent for secondary analysis was not taken.

In situations wherein it is impractical and there are only minimal risks, requirements to obtain the informed consent of research participants may be waived, although a review by an EC is a necessary safeguard.[18] For example, in the case of some epidemiological studies and surveillance programs that involve the linkage of large databases that need regular compilation and maintenance for other purposes, it is not feasible to obtain the informed consent of individuals. In such circumstances, confidentiality safeguards and other measures must be employed so that there are no harmful outcomes from the intended research. Also, in an epidemiologic investigation on disease outbreaks or program evaluations as part of public health practice, informed consent requirements may be lessened or waived off. However, even in an outbreak investigation, it is often desirable and feasible to disclose the information on the purpose of the investigation. Consent from the community leaders or the local authorities who are normally responsible for their well-being could be taken to assure the participants.

To collect valid data with rigorous scientific principles applied to improve clinical care and public health interests, there have been guidelines from many countries for waiving off the need for consent forms. These guidelines mainly consider two facts: (1) impractical to administer/get consent and (2) minimal risk research.[18] It is impractical to get the consent of a participant who is dead, cannot be located/contacted, or the data which is desired to be reviewed is anonymized. Observational studies have been regarded as minimal-risk studies since they do not involve any procedures or administering any drug or device and that the risks involved are not over and above those encountered routinely. The review of clinical records and survey data is also seen as a minimal risk to the participant if the information is identifiable. However, RCTs could never be considered to have minimal risks, since participants are allotted to different intervention arms. Investigators have raised concerns for the lack of generalizability of results where selection biases have cropped in due to large numbers of nonconsenters. The anonymization of data makes it difficult to ensure that there is no duplication of individuals and to follow them up indirectly. The usefulness of obtaining informed consent from all the participants in the Registry of the Canadian Stroke Network and its impact on the generalizability of the results revealed that due to the selection biases, the registry patients were not representative of the typical patients with stroke at each participating center.[19] It also showed huge costs involved in consent-related processes. There are concerns with the definitions and perceptions across different populations and settings concerning minimal risks and impractical consent, and highlights for ECs to keep this in mind.

There has been agreement on waiver of consent in emergency/disaster/calamity care and research given the complexities involved in obtaining informed consent (first hand or proxy) and the need to develop better management strategies.[20] It is an ethical dilemma when individual rights are pitted against societal needs and physician's paternalism.

It is suggested that instead of the usual bulky and too technical informed consent and its procedure, ECs could allow "improvisation" in the content and usage of a local culturally suitable style of language/dialect to safeguard the rights and welfare of the participants. Community consultation and approvals would strengthen these measures.

Protecting the Welfare of Research Participants

Epidemiologists must abstain from conducting studies that may injure or jeopardize the welfare of the study participants by intentional or unintentional behaviors or actions (e.g., neglect or unjustified change from the EC approved study protocols or standards of practice) or omissions. The investigators must pay attention to psychological, economic, legal, or social risks and not limit to physical risks as a result of direct contact with participants.[1]

Most of the participants may not understand the concept of "risk" and "benefit" of participating in research. Inability to present the study in a balanced manner could weigh it more toward either risk or benefits. It becomes aggravated in the presence of poor understanding of the study participants. The blind faith in doctors and other health professionals makes them believe against any risk of participation.[7]

The dilemma is to define whether the consent form is referring to risk and benefit to the individuals alone, or the implications of research study to the society or community, which they represent. The results of individuals can have severe influences on their communities by way of stigmatization, like the results on the prevalence of mental disorders, high-risk behaviors, etc. When community-level consent for recruiting participants is being obtained, the risks and benefits for both should be made explicitly clear so that an informed decision for participation can be taken. The infamous experiment conducted from 1932 till 1972 on African-American males living in the town of Tuskegee, Alabama, USA, to study the natural history of latent syphilis, highlights racial discrimination and stigmatization of blacks. Several males with the infection died due to syphilis or progressed into the late stage of illness due to lack of treatment, despite the availability of Penicillin for therapy in the 1940s. The exposure of this study by a journalist led to the setting up of the National Commission for the Protection of Human Subjects of Biomedical and Behavioral Research. Similar concerns have arisen in researching seronegative partners of HIV-positive participants, to study the development of HIV in them. Informing the partners of HIV positivity would make them take precautions, which could most likely influence the study adversely. By not informing them, preventable and unnecessary exposure to HIV would occur which should alert the investigator to avoid such instances. Studies looking at racial or ethnic differences and their relationship to income, education, socioeconomic status, could lead to discrimination in employment, housing, or insurance. It also lowers the individual's self-esteem or the community eroding their cultural pride. Generalizing findings to a particular community or group should be avoided for example, generalizing that promiscuous homosexual men and long-distance truck drivers in developing countries are more likely to be HIV positive compared to chaste or monogamous people. This stigmatization caused difficulty to truck drivers in their state of residence (India) for getting married to girls in their area.[21] Similarly, the statement that nonresident Asians are at a greater risk of developing coronary artery disease is likely to stigmatize that community.[22] In situations wherein the disclosure of results must also provide information about the participant's geographical location/area, care must be taken to not imply any sort of moral criticism of the obtained participant's response/information.

These issues can be tackled by using appropriate ethical standards. It is challenging to undertake epidemiological studies in those populations or sections of the society, which are already disadvantaged. One has to balance the need to obtain accurate health information against the repercussions that the population would face given the findings. Additional ethical safeguards need to be put in place.

In long-term follow-up studies, there is a need to constantly balance and review the need to minimize sample size attrition (retain the participants, since they have the liberty to withdraw their participation from the study at any point of time without assigning any reason) with a humane instinct to offer health advice, especially if it is requested for. In a long-term study on the determinants of childhood obesity, a cohort of children was followed up since birth and their various physical and biochemical parameters were periodically recorded.[23] This study raised an issue concerning risks of participation, as to when does it become ethically necessary to offer health promotion advice or intervention to avoid the participant shifting from "normal" to "high-risk" category. These issues may hinder the epidemiologist's quest to collect unbiased, valid, and high-quality data, which would answer an important question.

It is an important ethical prerequisite to offer counseling and undertake follow-up based upon the need. It has been emphasized on several occasions that the study investigator cannot offer or deliver any intervention or treatment for the problems not covered in the study course of data collection that did not primarily aim at medical and psychological treatment. There is a moral obligation to provide the necessary care in such circumstances. Although treatment of emotional problems may be in the best interest of the child, parents may sometimes resent any intrusion of the researchers beyond simply conducting the research.

Investigators have argued that the research budget should include the cost of such counseling.

The data-collection methods such as questionnaires have been looked upon as risk-free, as the likely impact of questionnaires upon patients is not often considered and the balance of benefit and harm has not been fully explored.[24] Some evidence demonstrates that simply asking questions may become an active intervention similar to the administration of any physical treatment. This might also have the potential for psychological consequences of varied nature (e.g., increased anxiety). There is a need for the provision of robust consent procedures that can anticipate and confront the possible harms that can arise for all stakeholders—participants, practitioners, and investigators.

An epidemiological study undertaken in a developing country may have unique concerns; it can create the impression in the concerned community that they will be provided with health care, at least while the research workers are present. Thus, the disadvantaged populations are vulnerable to such expectations, while it is likely that the short- and long-term benefits may not reach them in their perceived quantum. Research groups "adopt" some of these populations to undertake long-term studies on risks and their outcomes. Assurance of providing ongoing healthcare benefits by them beyond the requirement of the research questions may be viewed as inducement at the population level since it tempts people to participate in anticipation of their overall well-being. While this could be considered reasonable inducement, it enables recruitment and follow-up of participants easier as trust builds between the participants and the investigators. Maintaining this trust becomes important for the investigators to accomplish the objectives from such populations.[25]

Equipoise denotes an investigator's genuine uncertainty concerning which arm or group is more likely to benefit from a clinical trial. It is not always possible for epidemiologists to be able to prevent all risks incurred by the study participants. For instance, clinical trials may pose greater risks (or benefits) for participants in the trial treatment or intervention arm than to those in the control or placebo arm (or vice versa).[25] Thus, before initiating the study the epidemiologists must ensure that the risks incurred on the participants (intervention arm) are reasonable and are in line with the anticipated benefits. Several meta-analyses have established that something (e.g., a patient education program) is always better and comes handy than nothing (e.g., usual care with no intervention). In conducting community-based RCTs in vulnerable/disadvantaged population, an ethical dilemma arises in assigning controls to the "usual care" group (which is usually substandard to the best care or the intervention arm). The disadvantaged population may like its entire people to be part of the "intervention arm" under the assumption that "new" intervention will be better than "usual care" since evidence suggests that the former would be better than the latter intervention. This leaves the researchers responsible to find an optimal balance between scientifically rigorous studies, pragmatic and operational feasibility, and associated ethical dilemmas. After a reasonable period of study, the "usual-care" group should get the intervention if it is proven to be more beneficial instead of prolonging the study further.

Vulnerable Groups in Epidemiological Studies

The vulnerability could include people with reduced autonomy, for example, cognitive or communicative disability (e.g., young children), institutionalized status (imprisonment), dependable (i.e., able to consent but subjugated to the authority of someone else), medical (having a serious ailment), economic (poor section of society), social (underprivileged social groups), and exposed to devastating conditions like natural and manmade disasters/calamities (earthquakes, poisonings, floods, etc.).[26]

Four critical areas of importance in the planning and conduct of research after a disaster include: (1) Decision-making capacity of the participant, (2) vulnerability, (3) risks and benefits in participation, and (4) informed consent. Major contributions have been made in enhancing knowledge, services, and outcomes for countless victims and their families by the research community, which has focused their attention in assessing and minimizing the impact of terror and disaster on affected individuals and communities. This research community can continue to serve the victims and survivors of traumatic events by maintaining sensitivity to the needs of this population. Also, there is a need to understand more on the effects of trauma and trauma-focused research participation along with pursuing their significant work.[27,28]

It should be assumed that, as a group, individuals affected by a disaster have the inherent capacity to provide meaningful and voluntary informed consent to participate in the research. It is not necessary to consider the disaster-affected populations as "vulnerable" in the regulatory sense. When any questions arise, then individual-level assessments must be conducted. There are capacity assessment tools available to be utilized for the purpose; however, they need to be monitored with time. The level of risk from the research determines the level of concern on the individual participant's capacity to consent. The willingness or decision to participate is completely dependent on the competent prospective participant.

There is always a need for additional research on the risks and benefits of participation in disaster-related research. Hence, specific research proposals must be critically scrutinized on the level of risk, the research novelty, and the uncertainty of the risk–benefit ratio. Such scrutiny may result in the need for further procedural safeguards. It is important to even study the effects incurred from the research on participants and if their expectations during the enrollment process were similar to the experience of participation.

Even in disturbing situations such as a disaster/calamity, representatives of the community, i.e., participants of the research, can have a certain level of involvement in the research planning and implementation. Information for potential research participants should clearly distinguish between therapeutic and research intent.

However, the provisions for the confidentiality of the data and protection of the privacy of the participants remain an integral part of the research plan. Thus, the groundwork for initiating disaster-related research should be in a safe, controlled environment that is conducive to making an informed decision about participation.

No compromises are allowed in explicit plans for the training and support of research staff who are exposed to the emotional challenges faced by research participants. Like in other epidemiological studies, the study participants in post-disaster research must be informed about the results of the concerned research study. To enhance and minimize participant burden, coordination and collaboration among researchers and ECs may help. Also, various models can be considered to facilitate such coordination without unduly impeding research.

Of concern in psychiatric patients and other vulnerable groups such as children and those with intellectual impairment is the fact that they are difficult than others to engage and maintain for treatment and follow-up. A simpler and practical process for consenting would be useful in such situations. It can be argued that until research offers a level playing field with "adequate representation" of all groups, it will be failing the health needs of those it aims to serve.

Ethical guidelines advise that for research involving children and adolescents, consent for participation is obtained from their parents or legal guardians. A balance between legality and self-autonomy needs to be deliberated in such instances. The custodians of this vulnerable group desist from allowing them to participate as research participants, causing low response rates and poor scientific validity. Discussions have focused on the dilemma of how to promote the best interests of children as a group through research while protecting the rights and welfare of individual research participants. There exist multiple concerns in youth surveys, regarding: (1) who can give consent for children's participation in research, (2) how "informed" informed consent must be, (3) how to ensure that the information is understood by the differently abled children, (4) how to conduct surveys among abused children who might be emotionally harmed by being questioned about their experiences, and (5) how to provide information on study results when abuse is often unacknowledged.[29] Proxy consent is obtained to protect the interests of the participant; however, this does not express the person's autonomy since she/he has none or limited autonomy at that time. The issue of parents/guardians' refusal to consent to their children's participation in community surveys may pose concerns to even those studies on nonsensitive issues. Also, requiring parental consent can significantly lower participation rates. In a study, participants acknowledged that such a survey would be difficult to implement if it requires parental consent.[29]

Privacy and Confidentiality

Privacy refers to the individual's choice to be left alone and not forced into participating in the study, or participating on her/his terms, or withdrawing in between without assigning reasons. Confidentiality is preventing disclosure of information in ways that are inconsistent with the understanding under which the information was obtained. Individuals' privacy and confidentiality of information need to be ensured unless there is an overriding moral concern (e.g., health or safety) or requirement of law justifying the release of such information. If privacy or confidentiality must be breached, the epidemiologist should first attempt to inform participants of such required infringements.[1] In the event of disclosing information, agreement on whom to disclose, whether the participant is to be informed, how much information is to be disclosed, and whether the participant must authorize the disclosure are all needed to be considered. The ethics review committees could scrutinize and satisfy themselves with the mechanisms proposed by the investigator/sponsor in ensuring privacy and confidentiality, particularly in long-term follow-up studies.

Recently, concerns about maintaining confidentiality in epidemic outbreaks and the inappropriate use of genetic information are rising, for example, using confidential genetic information to refuse someone employment or deny any health insurance.

The ethical aspect of contacting patients enrolled in studies in which information is required repeatedly is a relatively neglected area of discussion. In such instances, "ethical considerations should be paramount" and to do otherwise is not only unethical but could impair the quality of information, since a "coerced" patient may provide less accurate data than a cooperative one.[16] Problems are further compounded, if the number of patients completing any scientific inquiry is too low to draw precise conclusions, or the withdrawals result in biased conclusions. In these cases, the studies themselves may become unethical, as the claims in the initial consent procedures to ask participants to engage in a scientific inquiry that will enhance knowledge are vitiated. Because of this, attempts are often made in both RCTs and other epidemiological studies that require periodic follow-up to improve the contact rate in various ways using the initial consent of the patient to access information systems and obtain other information. For example, telephone numbers, to maintain contact and overcome potential difficulties (such as change of address), changing names (getting married), and changing work patterns (shift work) could impair contact at times of planned assessment. Although this approach, best termed "anticipated consent" or "implied consent" as it is moving forward in time, has merits and certainly aids follow-up rates, it can also pose ethical difficulties. While this may be feasible for the initial phases of a trial, it would be very difficult to achieve in a study that involves follow-up at some time in the distant future.[16]

Participants of epidemiological studies should be advised that it may not always be possible to inform them of findings that pertain to their health, but they should not take this to mean that they are free of the disease or condition under study.[30] It may not be possible to often extract information on individuals and their families from pooled findings. When epidemiological data are unlinked, a disadvantage to participants is that individuals at risk cannot be informed of useful findings on their health. Under these circumstances, the ethical duty to do good can be served by making pertinent healthcare advice available to their communities.

This is relevant to arguments about the merits of "cold calling," the practice of calling people (occasionally in person) who have not formally agreed to take part in a research investigation but who have not actively refused either or, in some cases, have given anticipated consent.[16] It is argued that those who disapprove of such a practice as a possible infringement of liberty by such assertive behavior, particularly when it is not accompanied by any benefit to the individuals concerned, the nonresponse to an invitation to be interviewed in such an instance should be interpreted as a passive refusal. An alternative view is that many who do not respond to letters or other forms of inquiry have genuinely expressed no opinion and therefore are open to further invitations. When these are taken together, the second may take precedence over the first in the search for more complete data that enables more precise conclusions to be drawn. At each follow-up interview, if circumstances change, then consent needs to be re-obtained (fresh or re-consent). It may also be argued that cold calling is ethical in the context of long-term, follow-up studies provided that coercion is prevented.

Issues of patient confidentiality can hamper epidemiological research. A wider debate is required about the use of medical records to identify eligible individuals. ECs need to consider the benefits to society against ethical dilemmas of diverse natures when debating and discussing studies. The use of public funds should be considered as part of the cost to society if a study cannot recruit participants by the most effective and valid methods. The National Creutzfeldt–Jakob Disease Surveillance Unit of the UK desired to recruit controls to study the risk factors for the variant form of the disease from the community from which the cases were detected.[31] The local practitioners who had reported the cases were requested to identify randomly 20 relatives of controls from their practice and send them letters regarding their permission to be approached by the surveillance team investigators. The low response rates (16%) for agreeing to participate and their selection bias limited the validity of the study. Aggressive measures such as approaching the participants directly by the investigators raised concerns as this was seen as a breach of confidentiality.

For certain epidemiological studies, selective or partial disclosure may be benign and ethically permissible. However, it should not induce participants to do what they would not otherwise consent to do. An Ethics Review Committee may permit disclosure of only selective information when this course is justified. This is especially relevant in some RCT studies and decisions taken in public health interest. To achieve the targets of polio eradication from India, a list of families who were resistant to give polio drops to their young children was made available to researchers to facilitate studies on sociocultural determinants of resistance. The families were surprised that their names were accessible and known beyond their area of residence—is that stigmatization? However, the reports were anonymized so that the community/families/individuals were not identifiable.

With the advancements in information technology, legal frameworks and professional guidance must be created or refined to safeguard the rights of patients. To facilitate future research, it should be ensured that sufficient mechanisms are in place to inform patients about any potential use of their data for research and trust is built to obtain consent when necessary. Finally, researchers should discuss well in advance their project design with those responsible for data protection and data audit and accordingly arrive at a consensus. On the other hand, ECs and investigators should consider selective disclosure for the larger public good and changing societal as well as individual needs. These should be guided by the prevailing regulations, statutory requirements, and guidelines in place.

Sociocultural Contexts of Research

Disruption of social mores is usually regarded as harmful. Cultural values and social mores must be respected. It may be a specific aim of an epidemiological study to stimulate change in certain customs or conventional behavior to lead to healthier behaviors, for example, diet or a hazardous occupation. Although members of communities have a right not to have others impose an uninvited "good" in them, those studies expected to result in health benefits are usually regarded as ethically acceptable and not harmful. Healthy and open-minded discussions with community leaders and other stakeholders are desirable. Investigators must ensure not to overstate the benefits to unduly influence a community's agreement to participate. Investigators must respect the standards of ethics being followed in that setting and the cultural expectations of the societies when investigating cultural groups different from their own in which the study is being undertaken.

Distributive justice is an important aspect of ethical practices. All persons and groups must be treated equally, though the equal distribution of benefits and burdens may be modified by considerations of special need or merit. For instance, vulnerable classes of persons in society and those in special need may merit additional benefits (while bearing fewer burdens). The potential benefits of epidemiology should extend to all groups of persons in society including those who are socioeconomically disadvantaged.

Since the consent form is seen more as a document with legal implications, people hesitate to sign it. It should be seen within the particular contexts of regional values and practices, local concepts of disease and health, power hierarchies in the family and the community, and the socio-cultural milieu.[7] The understanding that similar interpretations of ethical principles are applicable cross-culturally may not be valid.[8]

Ethics Review

Irrespective of the source of the proposals—academic, governmental, health care, commercial, or others—it is a prerequisite that proposals for epidemiological studies be submitted to ethics review. Sponsors must be able to identify the necessity of ethics review and facilitate the establishment of ethics review committees. Studies undertaken during emergencies (disasters or calamities) must be submitted for ethics review since the participants are likely to be vulnerable. The need for social distancing, nationwide lockdown, and quarantine during the COVID-19 pandemic has led the community to face a more vulnerable situation. In this scenario, the ECs play a very important role in reviewing protocols prepared for such emergency(s) and also ongoing non-COVID-19-related projects. It includes the use of expedited or fast-track processes but must ensure robust ethics review followed by monitoring the conduct of research. It is recommended to avoid face-to-face meetings and instead organize virtual conferences to observe social-distancing norms without compromising the scientific integrity along with protecting the rights, safety, and well-being of research participants. It is explained in detail in Section 3 of The National Guidelines for Ethics Committees reviewing Biomedical and Health Research during COVID-19 pandemic.[32]

Many authors have commented on the difficulties experienced by researchers in obtaining Ethics Committee approval for multicentric studies. These have been related mainly to tedious and unclear administrative requirements; high costs incurred by investigators to meet requirements; miscommunications amongst researchers of sites, central research ethics committees, and local ethical research committees; delays in approval time and timely commencement of research activities; and local changes which influence the response rates. These factors threaten the validity of the entire study and the generalizability of the results.[33] The problems researchers have with multicenter research are often structural and logistic and not due to substandard working of local research ECs. However, attempts by all concerned are to be made to bring more coordination between local and federal research ECs through timely submission of protocols. The realization that multicentric studies have more impact on practice guidelines, policy, and program planning requires extra efforts on the part of the ECs in their review process. During the course of the study, any changes made to the protocol requires re-approval from the Ethics Committee.[14]

There are three major public health activities with ethical concerns: surveillance activities, emergency response, and program evaluation.[26] All these activities involve data collection to improve disease treatment, prevention, and control. The information can be used to look for its use in similar settings elsewhere also. The definitions and concepts have been elucidated in several places, but the common dilemma concerns their requirement for ethical review and its processes. Public health could involve research and nonresearch activities aimed at societal levels. The key difference between the two lies in the intent to undertake the activity, whether it is to generate information on human participants that can be generalized or data being collected for disease prevention and control in the identified population. Hence, all activities which have research intent, whether at the beginning of the activity or later on, will require ethics review. It is difficult to have a common prescription for all activities; instead, they have to be considered on a case-to-case basis. Local guidelines must be made available to public health professionals and other investigators.

Most ECs are unable to differentiate public health activities versus epidemiological research and thus apply the same ethical principles. This raises issues related to individual's rights versus public benefits. Program evaluation activities will also require ethics review by the full committee since they are likely to influence a large population, which could include vulnerable sections of society. This also provides a review of the scientific vigor of the proposal by the full committee.

Public Trust

Public trust is essential for any of the epidemiologic functions such as disease surveillance, outbreak investigations and control, and research. Trust is an expression of faith and confidence that the investigators will be fair, reliable, ethical, competent, and nonthreatening. However, if epidemiologists perceive that a health problem exists but is being ignored or its existence denied by the community, then it is appropriate to proceed with a study of a health problem (or an outbreak investigation that must be initiated without delay to address an urgent public health concern) while simultaneously working with the community to gain their confidence and support.

To promote public trust, power dynamics should be considered especially in communities with reduced power. In such an instance, epidemiologists must adopt a "participatory" approach for designing their research and ensuring care that community participation does not adversely affect scientific objectivity. The establishment of a community advisory board may be helpful to oversee and guide the research team. When planning and conducting occupational epidemiology studies, it is always desirable to obtain inputs from workers or their representatives. It will be a challenge for the investigator to obtain informed trust from the community, which does not lead to inducements. It will generally be possible if the scientific facts and motives of the study are put forth in a simple, transparent, and nonpartisan manner.[34]

Conflicts of Interest

The epidemiological studies undertaken during outbreaks, epidemics, disasters, and calamities by providers of relief and rehabilitation can have a conflict of interest and/or indulge in unethical practices. Relief workers providing relief on one hand also become an instrument for conducting research. The free will and voluntary participation of victims will likely be jeopardized, even if they would have wanted to do so. In occupational and environmental health fields, several well-defined special interest groups may conflict. In such situations, it may be difficult to avoid pressures from such conflicts of interest and thus can lead to distorted interpretations of study results. The ethics review committees must be sensitive to these risks of conflict. They should not approve proposals with any such inherent conflict of interest except in those disclosed to prospective participants and their communities.

Obligations to Communities

Epidemiologists meet their obligations to communities by undertaking public health research. They undertake related activities that can address the causes of morbidity and mortality or studies on utilization of healthcare resources. Timely reporting of such study results is beneficial to address the community needs. Epidemiologists must carefully consider any premature and unnecessary delay in the release of research findings. The research findings must be interpreted and made available to the public following the current scientific knowledge concurrent to their utility and validity. Appropriate peer review, replication, and other safeguards to assure scientific validity are important, but they require time. The under- or overstatement of the significance of findings of the study may almost construe to inaccurate information. The epidemiologists should upfront their study strengths and limitations (research methods) in a legible perspective. There may be occasions when it becomes imperative to terminate a study early and release its findings to protect the public's health; such early terminations should occur only after due consultation with scientific peers, ethics review committees, and the study's oversight committee. Also, reasons for the early release of results must be clearly articulated in every instance.

Epidemiologists have to strive that research findings are interpreted and reported accurately and appropriately as they cannot always prevent the media or other parties from sensationalizing research results. The results of studies in progress leaked to the media or others can jeopardize the scientific integrity of the study or mislead the public and are likely to breach the privacy and confidentiality of the participants. The advocacy of the results can be a joint exercise of the sponsor and researcher since most investigators may not be in a position to take the results to the appropriate forum.

Epidemiologists must respect the diversities in culture when undertaking research, practice activities, and communicating with community members.[26] This can be ensured by being well-informed about the history, circumstances, perspectives, and group dynamics within the community.

CONCLUSION

There is widespread recognition of ethical issues surrounding epidemiological studies. The responsibility and accountability of researchers and ethics committees toward communities they belong are more explicitly understood now. However, societies are dynamic structures and ethical issues and their emerging concerns need constant thinking in light of new information and requirements. There is a need for constant debate and discussions among a range of stakeholders within the socio-cultural milieu of the intended research. Additional issues that need attention include ethical principles and standards of practice for the long-term retention of data in data archives and data audit, ethical issues arising in genetic research, consideration of the broader social and environmental consequences of epidemiologic research, and human rights considerations relevant to epidemiology. Not at the least, the society will have to constantly find a healthy equilibrium between ethics and the potential of robust scientific enquiry and innovations.

REFERENCES

1. American College of Epidemiology Ethics Guidelines. Ann Epidemiol. 2000;10(8):487-97.
2. Mahmood SS, Levy D, Vasan RS, Wang TJ. The Framingham Heart Study and the epidemiology of cardiovascular disease: a historical perspective. Lancet. 2014;383(9921):999-1008.
3. Central Drugs Standard Control Organization, Directorate General of Health Services, Ministry of Health & Family Welfare, Government of India. New Drugs and Clinical Trials Rules 2019 G.S.R. 227(E). New Delhi: CDSCO; 2019. [online] Available from: https://cdsco.gov.in/opencms/export/sites/CDSCO_WEB/Pdf-documents/NewDrugs_CTRules_2019.pdf [Last accessed October, 2021].
4. Beauchamp TL, Childress JF. Principles of Biomedical Ethics. New York: Oxford University Press; 1979.
5. Council for International Organizations of Medical Sciences (CIOMS) in collaboration with the World Health Organization (WHO). International Ethical Guidelines for Epidemiological Studies. CIOMS, Geneva: 2009. [online] Available from: https://cioms.ch/wp-content/uploads/2017/01/International_Ethical_Guidelines_LR.pdf [Last accessed October, 2021].
6. Scott CK, White WL. Ethical issues in the conduct of longitudinal studies of addiction treatment. J Subst Abuse Treat. 2005;28(Suppl 1):S91-S101.
7. DeCosta A, D'Souza N, Krishnan S, Chhabra MS, Shihaam I, Goswami K. Community based trials and informed consent in rural north India. J Med Ethics. 2004;30(3):318-23.
8. Angiolillo AL, Simon C, Kodish E, Lange B, Noll RB, Ruccione K, et al. Staged informed consent for a randomized clinical trial in childhood leukemia: impact on the consent process. Pediatr Blood Cancer. 2004;42(5):433-7.
9. Bhutta ZA. Beyond informed consent. Bull World Health Organ. 2004;82(10):771-7.
10. Wood, Susan Y, Friedland BA, McGrory CE. Informed consent: From good intentions to sound practices—A report of a seminar. In: Robert H (Ed). Ebert Program on Critical Issues in Reproductive Health Publication Series. New York: Population Council; 2002. p. 53.
11. Angus VC, Entwistle VA, Emslie MJ, Walker KA, Andrew JE. The requirement for prior consent to participate on survey response rates: a population-based survey in Grampian. BMC Health Serv Res. 2003;3(1):21.
12. Coiera E, Clarke R. e-Consent: The design and implementation of consumer consent mechanisms in an electronic environment. J Am Med Inform Assoc. 2004;11(2):129-40.
13. Elgesem D. What is special about the ethical issues in online research? Ethics Inf Technol. 2002;4:195-203.
14. Indian Council of Medical Research. National ethical guidelines for biomedical and health research involving human participants. New Delhi: Indian Council of Medical Research; 2017. [online] Available from: https://ethics.ncdirindia.org/asset/pdf/ICMR_National_Ethical_Guidelines.pdf [Last accessed October, 2021].
15. Rogers WA. Ethical issues in public health: a qualitative study of public health practice in Scotland. J Epidemiol Community Health. 2004;58(6):446-50.
16. Tyrer P, Seivewright H, Ferguson B, Johnson T. "Cold calling" in psychiatric follow up studies: is it justified? J Med Ethics. 2003;29(4):238-42.
17. Al-Shahi R, Vousden C, Warlow C; Scottish Intracranial Vascular Malformation Study (SIVMS) Steering Committee. Bias from requiring explicit consent from all participants in observational research: prospective, population based study. BMJ. 2005;331(7522):942.
18. Lertsithichai P. Waiver of consent in clinical observational research. J Med Assoc Thai. 2005;88(2):275-81.

19. Tu JV, Willison DJ, Silver FL, Fang J, Richards JA, Laupacis A, et al. Impracticability of informed consent in the Registry of the Canadian Stroke Network. N Engl J Med. 2004;350(14):1414-21.
20. Richardson LD. The ethics of research without consent in emergency situations. Mt Sinai J Med. 2005;72(4):242-9.
21. Singh YN, Malaviya AN. Long distance truck drivers in India: HIV infection and their possible role in disseminating HIV into rural areas. Int J STD AIDS. 1994;5(2):137-8.
22. Ardeshna DR, Bob-Manuel T, Nanda A, Sharma A, Skelton WP 4th, Skelton M, et al. Asian-Indians: a review of coronary artery disease in this understudied cohort in the United States. Ann Transl Med. 2018;6(1):12.
23. Jeffery A, Snaith R, Voss L. Ethical dilemmas: feeding back results to members of a longitudinal cohort study. J Med Ethics. 2005;31(3):153.
24. Evans M, Robling M, Maggs Rapport F, Houston H, Kinnersley P, Wilkinson C. It doesn't cost anything just to ask, does it? The ethics of questionnaire-based research. J Med Ethics. 2002;28(1):41-4.
25. Anderson RM. Is it ethical to assign medically underserved African Americans to a usual-care control group in community-based intervention research? Diabetes Care. 2005;28(7):1817-20.
26. Thomas J. Introduction to Modules 3 and 4: Research Ethics in Public Health. In: Jennings B, Kahn J, Mastroianni A, Parker LS (Eds). Ethics and Public Health: Model Curriculum. Washington DC: Association of Schools of Public Health; 2003. pp. 75-84. [online] Available from: https://aspph-wp-production.s3.us-east-1.amazonaws.com/app/uploads/2014/02/EthicsCurriculum.pdf [Last accessed October, 2021].
27. Sumathipala A, Siribaddana S. Research and clinical ethics after the tsunami: Sri Lanka. Lancet. 2005;366(9495):1418-20.
28. Collogan LK, Tuma F, Dolan-Sewell R, Borja S, Fleischman AR. Ethical issues pertaining to research in the aftermath of disaster. J Trauma Stress. 2004;17(5):363-72.
29. Helweg-Larsen K, Bøving-Larsen H. Ethical issues in youth surveys: potentials for conducting a national questionnaire study on adolescent school children's sexual experiences with adults. Am J Public Health. 2003;93(11):1878-82.
30. Al-Shahi R, Warlow C. Using patient-identifiable data for observational research and audit. BMJ. 2000;321(7268):1031-2.
31. Ward HJT, Cousens SN, Smith-Bathgate B, Leitch M, Everington D, Will RG, et al. Obstacles to conducting epidemiological research in the UK general population. BMJ. 2004;329(7460):277-9.
32. Indian Council of Medical Research. National Guidelines for Ethics Committees Reviewing Biomedical & Health Research During COVID-19 Pandemic. New Delhi: Indian Council of Medical Research; 2020. [online] Available from: https://ethics.ncdirindia.org//asset/pdf/EC_Guidance_COVID19.pdf [Last accessed October, 2021].
33. Tully J, Ninis N, Booy R, Viner R. The new system of review by multi-centre research ethics committees: prospective study. BMJ. 2000;320(7243):1179-82.
34. TRUST. Global Code of Conduct for Research in Resource-Poor Settings (2018). Available from: https://www.globalcodeofconduct.org/wp-content/uploads/2018/05/Global-Code-of-Conduct-Brochure.pdf [Last accessed October, 2021].

CHAPTER 5

Research Ethics in Participants with Mental Illness

Sunita Simon Kurpad

ABSTRACT

As persons with mental illness (PMI) are a vulnerable group, it is vital that all involved in mental health research are aware of the ethical issues involved. Following the letter and the spirit of the Indian Council of Medical Research (ICMR) National Ethical Guidelines for research involving human participants will ensure that ethical research is done in PMI too. All researchers as well as ethics committee (EC) members need to understand why participants with mental illness and their caregivers are considered to be a vulnerable group. Mental illnesses constitute a diverse group of illnesses, some of which have a relapsing course. The personal integrity of the researcher is paramount. However, as participants and caregivers will not automatically grasp that the researcher–participant relationship is not the same as the doctor–patient relationship, the onus is on researchers and research proposal reviewers to ensure that systems are in place to protect the rights and safety of participants. In this chapter, issues ranging from the diagnosis of mental illness; informed consent when the capacity to make the judgment about participation in a study is impaired; benefit-risk assessment around design of certain types of studies; voluntariness; the role of nominated representatives; psychiatric research in the COVID-19 pandemic; and other relevant issues are discussed.

INTRODUCTION

Mental health issues, directly and indirectly, are among the leading causes of disability and mortality across the world including India.[1] In 2016, depressive disorders ranked number 13 in WHO's list of the global top 20 causes of DALYs (disability adjusted life years), accounting for 1.7% of the DALYs.[2] In India, it has been reported that 1 in 7 persons is affected by mental illness of varying severity. Mental disorders contribute to 4.7% of DALYs in India, with depressive disorders contributing to 33.8% of the DALYs due to mental disorders.[3] There is a need to generate and understand evidence on clinical, biological, social, and psychological aspects of mental illness, its treatment, and outcomes. This would make research in mental illness an ethical requirement as persons with mental illness (PMI) also need evidence-based healthcare.

Research involving PMI raises ethical issues, which are relevant to any participant of medical research—from confidentiality to post-research benefit sharing as discussed comprehensively in the ICMR guidelines.[4] In addition, most mental illnesses at certain time points of the course of the illness confer particular vulnerabilities to the PMI. The ICMR National Ethical Guidelines, 2017, recognize the vulnerability of individuals with mental illness in section 6.8[4] and in its Handbook, 2018, in section 6.9.[5] This chapter will discuss the research participant as the PMI, a vulnerable group in research, and some of the ethical challenges that could stem from certain fundamental aspects of mental illness. It is hoped this understanding will help both researchers and EC members to ensure that the participation of PMI in research will not lead to exploitation or violation of their human rights. Understanding how mental illness and its treatment impact ethical considerations is not to prevent research involving PMI, but rather to facilitate ethical research involving them, and thus not discriminate against them.

THE ROLE OF NATURE OF ILLNESS, ITS COURSE, AND SETTING OF RESEARCH

Mental illness covers a spectrum of disorders. The ethical issues raised in a person with a psychotic illness would be different from that with a mood disorder, substance use or personality disorders. This would again be different if the person is acutely symptomatic, improving or in remission (in psychotic illnesses patients may experience a degree of disconnect with reality due to experiences, such as delusions and hallucinations). Participants may also have comorbid physical and other psychiatric illnesses. Sometimes, issues may be picked up on screening "normal" populations. This means that the ethical challenges faced by researchers in a psychiatric institution would be somewhat different from those faced in an outpatient clinic in a general hospital, in a community setting, in a rehabilitation center or in a college counselor's office. In addition, advances in mental healthcare have led to an improved prognosis and change in understanding about some mental illnesses. In addition to medications, there are ethical issues with the psychosocial interventions that are provided in mental healthcare.[6,7]

THE THREE CENTRAL AREAS OF VULNERABILITY

In PMI, three issues have long been recognized as particular concerns.[8] They are:
1. Ability of mentally ill participants of research to give an informed consent ("capacity")
2. Issues around the benefit–risk ratio
3. Voluntariness in providing the consent

Trained mental health professionals (which include clinical psychologists, psychiatric social workers, psychiatric nurses, trained occupational therapists as well as psychiatrists) will be aware of the issues around this vulnerability, as it is not fundamentally different from issues that arise during the clinical practice of psychiatry. This makes it particularly important to ensure that all research protocols also have a subject expert to review it, not just for the scientific validity, which is critical, but to also ensure that this vulnerability is not exploited, as can happen even inadvertently. While in the developed countries, some researchers have felt that ECs have overemphasized the specific vulnerability of PMI and been overly restrictive,[9] it is extremely important that everyone involved in research understands how the vulnerabilities in PMI can impact several arenas.

ARENAS OF ETHICAL CONCERNS

The following paragraphs will discuss some of the ethical aspects surrounding issues that impact research. These are not mutually exclusive, as one aspect can affect another.

The Diagnosis of Mental Illness

While the biological treatments of depression and anxiety disorders, or psychotic illnesses, such as schizophrenia and bipolar disorder, involve the use of medication that alters neurotransmitter levels or functioning, the diagnosis of mental illness is still based on the description of a constellation of symptoms and signs and the degree of distress and/or dysfunction experienced by the patient or by others due to the patient's behavior. While diagnostic criteria elucidated in WHO's ICD-10 (International Classification of Diseases, 10th revision) and American Psychiatric Association's DSM-5 (Diagnostic and Statistical Manual, 5th revision) are accepted as the gold standards in clinical care, improved understanding of what constitutes mental illness and what is not has led to diseases being included or excluded over time.[10,11] For example, in ICD-11, which is expected to be functional in January 2022, gaming addiction has been added, while gender incongruence has been taken out from the mental health section and placed in sexual health.[12]

We need to be aware that some PMI, early in the course of illnesses, may have a degree of denial, or a sense of stigma about their diagnosis. In India, a psychiatric diagnosis can impact issues ranging from marriage to job prospects. So, it would be best if the PMI are approached for recruitment into a study only with the permission of the treating psychiatrist and confidentiality strictly maintained.

In addition, while the clinical impression of trained psychiatrists using specific criteria may be used for research, validated scales, such as the Mini International Neuropsychiatric Interview (MINI PLUS), are generally used to generate diagnosis.[13] Sometimes research diagnostic criteria are used. Other scales that have been used in the past are Schedules for Assessment in Neuropsychiatry (SCAN) and the Composite International Diagnostic Interview (CIDI).

The MINI version 5.0, SCAN, and CIDI are based on ICD-10 and DSM-4, while MINI version 7.0 is based on new DSM-5.[13-16] It is important that the right person uses the right tool for the right purpose. For example, sometimes a scale used to screen for depression would be different from the one used to diagnose depression, while another one is used to measure its severity. This is important as some symptoms of mental illness, such as insomnia, anxiety, and feeling sad, can be part of the normal experience of life. Often it is the context, duration, severity of symptoms and dysfunction, which will distinguish normality from mental illness. The training of the person administering the scale is also important to address issues of reliability. While many scales are freely available, others are copyrighted. Researchers would need to check the usage rights, follow the process to either pay for the scales used or contact the publishers/copyright holder, and request a waiver (which is sometimes granted for small unfunded/low-funded studies). The ethical concerns about the medicalization of some behaviors, such as bereavement—the "medicalization of normality"[17] and the influence of pharmaceutical industry, place a greater ethical responsibility on researchers and EC members to ensure the measures used are appropriate to the research question. This is where a review by a subject expert in clinical practice would be additionally invaluable for the EC to arrive at a decision.

It would be useful to understand the meaning of certain terminologies and their context **(Table 1)**.

Informed Consent Process

The emphasis on informed consent is the bedrock on which one is able to ensure ethical research in medicine. Informed consent implies not only that all the relevant information has been given, but that the research participant has understood all of it and is able to make an informed decision as to whether to participate in the research or not. In PMI, the

TABLE 1: Meaning of terminologies and their context.

Terminology and context	Meaning
Mental illness—clinical practice of psychiatry	The clinical impression of psychiatrists, doctors or trained mental health professionals based on listing of illness and symptoms as per International Classification of Diseases 10th version (ICD-10) or Diagnostic and Statistical Manual-5 (DSM-5).[10,11]
Mental illness—research	Diagnosis generated by psychiatrists or trained professionals by using validated scales. The caveats with use of these scales need to be borne in mind, as already discussed in paragraph on diagnosis.
Mental illness—Mental Health Care Act, 2017 (MHCA)	"Mental illness" means a substantial disorder of thinking, mood, perception, orientation or memory that grossly impairs judgment, behavior, capacity to recognize reality or ability to meet the ordinary demands of life, mental conditions associated with the abuse of alcohol and drugs, but does NOT include mental retardation, which is a condition of arrested or incomplete development of mind of a person, especially characterized by subnormality of intelligence.[18] (Due to the negative connotations associated with the term "mental retardation", the term "intellectual disability" is now the more socially acceptable term.)
Person with disability (The Rights of Persons with Disability Act, RPWD Act, 2016)	Person with disability means a person with long-term physical, mental, intellectual or sensory impairment, which, in interaction with barriers, hinders his full and effective participation in society equally with others.[19]
Intellectual disability (The Rights of Persons with Disability Act, RPWD Act, 2016)	"A condition characterized by significant limitation both in intellectual functioning (reasoning, learning, problem solving) and in adaptive behavior which covers a range of everyday social and practical skills including specific learning disabilities and autism spectrum disorders"[19] (Note that the term mental retardation is not used here).
Cognition and cognitive impairment	Cognition broadly refers to our ability to think, understand, remember, and plan. It is a function of the brain and includes mental processes by which we acquire, retain, and use information. Cognition is critical in decision-making. While cognitive impairment is a broad term, it is often used to denote attention and memory difficulties.

challenge is in that some illnesses can fundamentally affect cognition—the ability to think, understand, remember, and plan **(Table 1)**, and this in turn will impact their capacity to give informed consent.

Cognitive Impairment and Capacity

Cognitive impairment can be due to a range of disorders, and can be temporary or permanent. For example, attentional difficulties in delirium or acute state of confusion can be due to physical disorders, such as alcohol withdrawal, from which persons can recover completely. Dementia can cause a cognitive decline with forgetfulness, which depending on the cause, may be permanent. Cognitive impairment can also occur with intellectual disability, while mental illnesses, such as depression and psychosis, can temporarily influence cognition. It is not only attention and memory that influences thinking and decision-making, but experiences like delusions (false beliefs) can also affect a PMI's ability to give an informed consent.[20]

The best way to practically ensure ethical recruitment into a study is to remember that assessing capacity and taking informed consent should not be a one-time event, but an iterative process.[21] Depending on whether the patient has the capacity to give informed consent or not, the correct process should be followed as given below:

- When the participant is capable of giving informed consent to participate in the study: In this situation, informed consent from participant (PMI) should be obtained. Generally, most PMI in India would have one or more trusted family members or a friend involved in their clinical care—a primary caregiver. While the choice to inform them or not about the research should reside with the PMI, the potential research participants should be encouraged to discuss it with them. Including a PMI, who does not want to inform any friend or family, into a research protocol needs to be carefully reviewed, as the issues of vulnerability may crop up later during the research. In India, unlike countries like the UK, healthcare is not routinely linked to a general health practitioner or a national health service, which would raise the question of who could be involved in taking care of the patient should the clinical need arise during research or should the PMI drop out during the research period or what happens after the research period. In addition, costs of healthcare are often borne by PMI and family. All this points to the fact that it would be important for researchers to document discussion with the PMI and key caregivers during the informed consent process. Sometimes researchers worry about giving all required details to the PMI. For example, in a randomized control trial (RCT), disclosing rare side effects of medication to a patient with depression or anxiety is difficult but nonetheless it has to be done. Informed consent refusals may be high, but some participants would still take part in the interests of science if they are convinced of the safety nets in place for the study.
- When the participant is not capable of giving informed consent to participate in the study: In certain illnesses like dementia or some intellectual disabilities, the

person may be unable to understand and process all the information given in order to make an informed decision about participation in research. In conditions like acute psychosis, this may be a temporary inability.

If a person is not able to give informed consent due to mental illness or cognitive impairment (*see* Table 1), it has been discussed in the section on vulnerability in ICMR National Ethical Guidelines (2017) that the informed consent of the legally authorized/acceptable representative (LAR) should be taken. ICMR National Ethical Guidelines for Biomedical Research in Children (2017) emphasize that in children the consent has to be taken from parents or the LAR stating that "a LAR is an individual or judicial or other body authorized under applicable law to consent on behalf of a prospective participant to participate in research or to undergo a diagnostic, therapeutic, or preventive procedure as per research protocol".[22]

As India had been a signatory to the United Nations Convention for the Rights of Persons with Disabilities (UNCRPD), there was an effort to ensure that the recent Mental Healthcare Act (MHCA) of 2017 was harmonized with the UNCRPD.[18,19,23] In the UN "Mental Health and Human rights" report by the High Commissioner for Human Rights at the UN General Assembly in 2017, the gap in research on mental health was noted. This was in the context of the discrepancy in valuing physical versus mental health, in particular to research on human rights aspects of mental healthcare.[24] However, it has been noted that (in principle) the Indian Mental Healthcare Act of 2017 has good concordance with WHO's checklist on mental health legislation on research.[25,26]

The Indian Mental Healthcare Act (MHCA, 2017) uses the term nominated representative (NR) for the person who is involved in "supported decision-making" when the capacity of the PMI to take decisions regarding own healthcare is affected. The entire Chapter IV of the MHCA is devoted to the definition of who can be construed as NR, the procedure for selecting the NR and their role. In principle, the PMI can nominate someone as their NR, as someone who can support them in making decisions. The MHCA specifies that the presence of a NR should not make one assume that the PMI does not have the capacity to make decisions. The term LAR as legally acceptable representative in the context of research described in ICMR National Ethical Guidelines of 2017 is not used in the MHCA, 2017.[18] However, the two terms NR and LAR are synonyms used for clinical care and research, respectively. If the PMI has not nominated an NR, the MHCA specifies an order of precedence of people who can be accepted as NR for the purpose of advance directives, as relative, caregiver, person appointed by the State Mental Health Board, and finally the Director of Social Welfare or their representative as appointed by the Board. For a minor (person with age <18 years), the legal guardian is considered to be the NR, unless a concern is communicated to the Board that the legal guardian is not acting in the best interest of the child or does not have the capacity to be the child's NR. In this situation, the Board will appoint a suitable person or appoint the Director of Social Welfare or their representative to act as NR. While the challenges in using NR in clinical care in India have been noted, it is probably easier when the primary caregiver is also the NR.[27]

Section 99 of the MHCA requires that several criteria be fulfilled before any interventional ("psychological, physical, chemical or medicinal" interventions) research can be undertaken if the PMI is incapable of giving informed consent.[18] These criteria include informed consent from the NR of the PMI, permission from the State Mental Health Authority; ethics approval from the EC where the research is going to be conducted; following all local, national, and international guidelines on ethical research; and declaration of no conflict of interest by researchers. The fundamental requirement should be that the research question is relevant and useful, and can *only* be answered by taking such patients into the study. And importantly, no research should be conducted if the PMI is unwilling for it. Even if the NR has given the informed consent for a PMI who is not capable of informed consent, no research activity should be performed if the PMI does not at least "assent" (as in "agree") to it, for example, to take a blood sample without the assent would amount to assault. On a practical level, to even ask questions for a rating scale, which involves cooperation, would not be possible if there is no assent. If the PMI is experiencing a condition like acute psychosis, then as soon as the patient's clinical condition improves and the patient becomes capable of giving informed consent that should also be taken (of course, assuming that the NR had "consented", as well as the PMI had "assented" at the start of the research). Like in any other research, the PMI and NR should be aware that they are free to withdraw their assent/consent at any time. It is important to follow the procedure as laid out by the prevailing law of the land to ensure that the rights of the PMI are protected, and ECs and research investigators do not get into difficulties later.

- Use of audio-visual recording of consent process: In the new regulations for clinical trials in India (New Drugs and Clinical Trials Rules, 2019), there is a requirement for audio-visual recording of the informed consent process when vulnerable patients are recruited for participation in a trial involving a new chemical or molecular entity.[28] While there could be understandable concerns about confidentiality, this step is considered necessary to ensure that the consent is truly informed and voluntary.

(Of course, the participant needs to consent to the audiovisual process too.) As there is a statutory requirement that study material be preserved for a certain number of years, investigators and ECs need to ensure that adequate steps are taken to protect the privacy of the data, including that of the audio-visual recording.

- The assessment of capacity to give informed consent: Mental illnesses encompass a range of disorders, which affect the thinking or cognition of persons differently (**see Table 1**). Lack of insight (awareness and acceptance that they have a mental illness) can also be a fundamental part of the experience of psychoses for some patients. In addition, insight can change during the course of illness and its treatment with relapse of illness or during the research period itself. There may not be a one-to-one relationship between insight and capacity. Capacity for informed consent in PMI is task- and time-specific. For example, a participant in partial remission of schizophrenia, who is still hearing voices, might be able to give informed consent to participate in a study that involves the use of rating scales to assess illness experience. However, a PMI in a manic episode is unlikely to have the judgment to understand the risks involved in a placebo control study. The PMI might know of the risks, but might feel it is not applicable to them, as being unduly confident can be part of the illness experience of mania.

Across the world, there are tools, such as MacCAT-CR (the McArthur assessment of competence tools for clinical research), which have been described for the assessment of decisional making capacity in schizophrenia.[21] As informed consent can be context driven, objective measures of insight and capacity might not always be useful.[29] If one is conducting research in acutely ill psychotic patients, some degree of diminished capacity might be inevitable. So it would be vital to get informed consent from the NR/LAR and the assent of the PMI, and follow the process laid down in the Mental Healthcare Act of India (2017) as described earlier.[30] In PMI with impaired decisional capacity, an iterative consent process using simple language to convey the participant information has been found to be useful.[21] Empirical research in India has shown that the capacity of the NR/LAR should not be presumed to be present. It would appear that assessment of the capacity of the NR/LAR who is giving proxy consent on behalf of the research participant is also warranted.[29] It has been suggested that the person who assesses capacity to consent should be independent of the research recruiting team.[31] It is possible that this might come across as logistically tedious in India, but it would be a good practice to avoid conflict of interest in the inclusion of PMI in research. This is particularly important till further evidence on matter of objective tests of capacity is available, as the clinical opinion of the treating mental health professional may be more useful in ascertaining if the PMI has the capacity to consent for a particular research study.

Benefit–risk Assessment

An RCT would be indicated only when there is clinical equipoise (i.e., a genuine uncertainty as to which treatment arm is better). Nearly 40 years ago, Helmchen and Müller-Oerlinghausen discussed an ethical dilemma in the "paradox of the clinical trial", summarizing the conundrum as "First, it is unethical to use treatment, the efficacy of which has not been tested scientifically; second, it is also unethical to examine the efficacy of treatment scientifically".[32] This need not be too much of a dilemma, if the pros and cons are understood and weighed carefully. "Therapeutic misconception" does exist, that is, participants tend to think the research would be of therapeutic benefit for them. It would obviously be important to ensure that the benefits and risks are clearly communicated both to the PMI and their caregivers and/or NR/LAR. In clinical interactions, trust in the doctor–patient relationship is important with many patients and caregivers understanding and expecting that clinicians take decisions in the patient's best interest. While the researcher is expected to conduct the research ethically, the researcher–participant relationship is not exactly the same as the doctor–patient relationship.[31] When researchers plan potentially risky protocols, such as an RCT with placebo control, wash out of treating medication or challenge studies where there is risk of precipitating mental illness[33], the PMI and family members may not fully appreciate the risk, despite it being written in the participant Information Sheet. While one would expect that participants are not wrong is trusting researchers, there should be adequate safety nets in place, which would be important for ECs to decide whether benefits outweigh risks and there are adequate procedures in place to detect risk situations, such as nonimprovement or early clinical worsening, in which case it will be ensured that the PMI will be taken out of the study and offered appropriate treatment.

The placebo trials in mental illness have invited criticism (and some support), both abroad and in India.[34] On one hand, it would arguably be unethical to offer placebo in illnesses where gold standard treatment is available, yet in some illnesses with a strong placebo response, some researchers feel it may be important to compare the new drug to a placebo. In July 2018, the World Medical Association adopted the Declaration of Helsinki (version amended in 2013). It has a paragraph on the use of placebo. It states that "The benefits, risks, burdens, and effectiveness of a new intervention must be tested against those of the best proven intervention(s), except in the following circumstances". It goes on to list these circumstances. These range from a situation where no proven intervention exists to ensure that patients who receive a less effective treatment should not experience irreversible or serious harm.[35] Those in favor of placebo control studies opine that it is methodologically superior, cheaper, and efficient due to the requirement of smaller sample sizes. Those against placebo control studies feel it violates the principle of equipoise when a standard treatment is available. They also feel it risks the deontological ethical principle as the possibility of benefit to society is at the risk of harm to a participant.[36] A detailed discussion of arguments for and against placebos would be outside the purview of this chapter, but readers could refer to the articles listed above. It is the considered opinion of this author that if placebo response data is available, and the protocol still proposes a comparison of a new drug (or old drug for a new indication) to a placebo, there should be a convincing reason as to why the comparison should not be to the gold standard treatment available. However, gold standards may have a lot of adverse events in comparison to the new drug. Another option would be to first compare the new drug to placebo to see if it is effective, or compare to placebo and the gold standard simultaneously. However, it would be important for EC reviewers not be influenced by stakeholders and be convinced for themselves about the ethics of the use of placebo or not in a particular study. What is important is that the use of placebo, method of randomization, and other relevant details are clearly discussed in the participant information sheet and informed consent form, in a language that the PMI and NR/LAR can understand. It would be important that the PMI and NR understand not only the potential risks/benefits but practical issues like the possibility of a longer stay in hospital if there is a nonresponse to placebo. The consent process should be clearly documented and witnessed.

Sometimes, the existence of independent Data safety and monitoring boards (DSMB) would be useful as its members are independent of the research team. It has also been pointed out that a default position of not allowing persons with severe mental illness to participate in research can be unhelpful because best practice evidence needs to be generated for that group too.[37]

Some Issues in Psychotherapy Research

There is evidence that placebo response not only occurs with medications, but also with medical interventions like procedures.[38] This would imply that the placebo response also needs to be accounted for in psychotherapy research. Sham interventions are one way of ascertaining placebo response in interventions. In order to perform a sham intervention arm of research ethically, it is important to inform the study participant *beforehand* that they could receive the sham treatment and get their consent.[39] The placebo response in psychotherapy exists, but is complex and challenging to measure.[40] Psychotherapy is sometimes studied alone, or in combination with medication. If controls like "waitlist controls" or "treatment as usual (TAU)" are used, its scientific validity and limitations should be borne in mind.[41] Informed consent in these situations should also include information about handling any undue distress while awaiting intervention/worsening of symptoms during the waitlist time, including accessing treatment/stopping participation in the study.

In the rare situation where an informed consent would undermine the rationale of the study, then ICMR Guidelines (point 5.11) discuss the role of deception in research and that EC may give permission with the consent as a two-stage procedure with a debriefing of the participant as soon as feasible.[4]

Researchers and EC members are also reminded that psychotherapy, while effective, is not immune to adverse effects.[42] Safety monitoring systems should be in place even for social and behavioral intervention studies.[43]

Voluntariness

Enthusiastic researchers may have blind spots in their drive/pressure to recruit patients. It is important that their enthusiasm does not result in or come across as coercion. The doctor–patient relationship is important in the care of a PMI as it has therapeutic value by itself and this needs to be protected. As the researcher–participant relationship is different, there could be a conflict of interest (COI) if the treating doctor is also a researcher involved in the study and tries to recruit the PMI into the study. This is yet another reason why it would be good practice to obtain the permission of the treating psychiatrist beforehand, as they might be in a good position to reiterate that if the PMI decides not to participate in the study, the doctor is not going to get annoyed and there would be no repercussions to their clinical care. The best way to ensure no COI is to ensure that one does not recruit patients under one's clinical care into one's own research. If that is impossible, at a minimum, someone else in the research team undertakes administration of the consent process and its documentation. This is particularly important in India as research has suggested that trust in the doctor and the institution can influence patients and family members to participate in clinical trials.[44]

Research in Relatively More Vulnerable Groups

It is important that researchers are made aware of PMI who are in relatively more vulnerable position like children and adolescents,[22,45] persons with substance use and high risk sexual behavior,[46] the elderly and prisoners among others. ICMR Guidelines for research in children[22] also mention about parents being particularly vulnerable to therapeutic misconception while consenting to their child's participation in research.

Post-research Benefit in Psychiatric Illnesses

This aspect of post-research benefit needs careful assessment by EC when reviewing research submissions. Psychiatric illnesses invariably need longer term treatment beyond the acute phase to reduce risk of relapse. This duration can last from 6 months to several years. It depends on various factors, for example, the nature of illness and past episode history. If the participant has responded best to the experimental drug, then changing or discontinuing the medication post-trial risks relapse. This can be a particular problem if there is delay in the drug being available in the market or is expensive. ICMR recommends in point 2.11.3 that EC ensures that these issues are discussed by the sponsor when the research is submitted for ethics consideration.[4]

Confidentiality and Data Privacy

Privacy of data is important and data should be stored and retrieved appropriately through controlled access.[47] Confidentiality has to be maintained unless information about a mandatorily reportable crime is obtained, for example, information pertaining to risk of homicide or the sexual abuse of minors as elucidated in the POCSO Act (Protection of Children from Sexual Offences Act), 2012. Retrospective research using case records need to be planned appropriately, needing EC approval for assured anonymity[48,18] and waiver of consent. An undertaking by the researcher should be submitted that the data will be anonymized by a third person.

Innovative Practices and Technological Advances in Psychiatry

The opinion of a mental health expert should be sought to ensure that the study is scientifically valid. This is particularly important in evaluating research using relatively newer methods, such as telepsychiatry, online therapy, app-based interventions, use of artificial intelligence, and other technological advances in psychiatry.

Some Ethical Issues with Use of the Internet

Ensuring privacy of research data is obviously important for any research, but it is particularly important in online mental health research due to the nature of the information requested.[49] As the internet is a public forum, both researchers and EC members need to consider steps such as data/email encryption and restricted access to data. The data security measures in place should be spelt out. As with any research, sometimes the participant's clinical condition can worsen and the need for specific intervention arise during the course of the study. Researchers need to be alert to adverse events, as they can occur with online interventions too. Safety nets in place to pick up "red flags" during online research and the process to refer such participants for intervention should also be clear.[50]

There are challenges in ensuring informed consent when there is no face-to-face interaction between the researcher and participant. If verbal consent is used, a script is advisable and signature of witness required. If information about the research and consent is being done online, steps to protect privacy should be taken and EC approval obtained before the study.[4] If cloud computing is likely and involvement of researchers across the globe, it would be important to know the terms of service providers and ensure there is no data access by others like advertisers. For work on "big data", the scientific and ethical pitfalls of use of algorithms and predictive models borne in mind. As the internet can be both a tool as well as a space for research, readers can access a more detailed discussion on the ethical challenges involved.[51] As technology evolves, so would the ethical and legal challenges. Till specific guidelines are available in India on this issue, readers might find the ethics guidelines for internet research brought out by the Association for Internet Researchers an additional useful resource.[52]

Research During Pandemic and Disaster Situations

In 2009, the WHO technical consultation on research ethics in international epidemic response highlighted the point that while the essence of the general principles of research ethics and protection of human rights remain the same in a public health emergency situation, there are some key differences.[53] EC members need to be alert to issues pertaining to changing perception of risk, benefits, need to "fast track" ethics review, yet ensure organizational accountability and transparency to ensure that substandard research or any unethical practices are flagged quickly.

In disaster situations, whether natural or man-made, the scale of healthcare requirements overwhelms the locally available resources. While mental stress can be understandable in these situations, it can precipitate mental illness in a vulnerable person or a person made vulnerable by extreme circumstances.

Research During the COVID-19 Pandemic

Research during the COVID-19 pandemic poses several additional challenges, both as a pandemic situation and, at times, a disaster situation. As discussing pandemic ethics and disaster ethics is beyond the scope of this section, readers are referred to WHO's training manual on this subject.[54] However, a few key points relevant to psychiatric research during the COVID-19 pandemic are briefly discussed below. The experience and lessons from the current COVID-19 scenario could be relevant to future epidemic/pandemic/disaster situations.

- *For continuing research started before the pandemic*: In view of the risks to participants and investigators due to travel or interaction with each other, the best action is to temporarily suspend research, till the risks subside. This would have to be discussed with the EC as well as the sponsors, if it is a funded study. As this could impact salaries of research investigators, it is important that everyone involved is kept informed of the uncertainty of the situation. If the study has to be prematurely stopped due to the COVID-19 situation, the impact on numbers recruited, and thereby the power of the study should be noted. Permissions from the EC for necessary amendments, validation of the online or telephone methodology/use of questionnaires should be done before proceeding further. If the research study could be continued with these modifications, then appropriate changes to the informed consent process for verbal or online consent should also be submitted to the EC.

- *For new research started during the pandemic*: From the evidence available till the moment this chapter goes to print, it seems possible that mental illness could be both a risk factor, as well as a complication of COVID-19.[55] In a position paper on COVID-19 and Mental Health, the need for good research practices even during the pandemic has been emphasized, including expedited reviews by ECs, the need for researchers to discuss protocols and questionnaires with patients/those with the lived experience, the need for harmonizing data/measures and global collaboration on the various aspects of mental health research ranging from neuropsychiatry to stigma.[56]

Additional Ethical Challenges in the COVID-19 Pandemic

Both researchers and ECs should keep in mind the fundamental ethical requirement that the research is truly needed and particularly valid during the COVID-19 pandemic. The fact that the pandemic has led to a glut of poor quality research[57] reminds us of the wisdom in Professor Doug Altman's words stated more than 15 years ago, "We need less research, better research and research done for the right reasons".[58] Online surveys can give useful information, if used correctly. Yet, the reality of the "digital divide" that many vulnerable persons will not be able to access online digital media should be borne in mind. One should not settle for poor quality data gathering merely because online surveys now seem easy to do, and some researchers feel the pressure to publish. If necessary, timelines may be fast tracked but scientific integrity and ethical requirements should never be compromised.[56] As discussed in the earlier section, "online" work with research participants (a fallout of the pandemic) requires that researchers and EC reviewers be alert to the ethical challenges surrounding privacy of data.

Research on Non-COVID-19-related Issues

For research on non-COVID-19-related issues during the pandemic, as reiterated earlier, relevant scientific questions should be addressed with appropriate methodology. But the additional requirement is to ensure the safety of research participants as well as research investigators.

Other General Relevant Issues

All other relevant ethical issues, which are relevant in research for persons without mental illness, are also obviously relevant in PMI. All COI should be declared, including any researcher–pharmaceutical company relationship. International collaborations including submissions to Health Ministry's Screening Committee (HMSC), genetic studies, storage of biological samples, insurance cover, contacting the PMI for future studies, and publication of research should all follow National Ethical Guidelines already available in this regard.[4,5,59]

CONCLUSION

This chapter discussed the various ethical issues that the researchers, reviewers, and EC members need to bear in mind while planning and conducting research in PMI. While PMI are a vulnerable group, there is a need to ensure good quality ethical research that will generate useful information on various aspects of mental health, mental illness, and its management. However, the most important "tool" to ensure ethical research is an ethical researcher. Personal integrity ensures safe research.[60,61] Till specific guidelines for PMI are available in India, researchers are also advised to additionally refer to the principles elucidated in the National Ethical Guidelines[4,5] and also addressed in international guidelines.[62]

REFERENCES

1. Institute of Health Metrics and Evaluation. India Datasets. [Online] Available from: http://www.healthdata.org/india [Last accessed October, 2021].
2. The Global Health Observatory. Global Health Estimates 2016: Disease burden by Cause, Age, Sex, by Country and by Region, 2000-2016. [Online] Available from: https://www.who.int/data/gho/data/themes/mortality-and-global-health-estimates.
3. India State-Level Disease Burden Initiative Mental Disorders Collaborators. The burden of mental disorders across states in India: the Global Burden of Disease Study 1990–2017. State Level Disease Burden Initiative Mental Disorders Collaborators. Lancet Psychiatry. 2020;7(2):148-61.
4. Indian Council of Medical Research (2017). National Ethical Guidelines for Biomedical and Health Research Involving Human Participants. [Online] Available from: https://ethics.ncdirindia.org/asset/pdf/ICMR_National_Ethical_Guidelines.pdf [Last accessed October, 2021].
5. Indian Council of Medical Research (2018). Handbook on National Ethical Guidelines for Biomedical and Health Research Involving Human Participants. [Online] Available from: https://ethics.ncdirindia.org/asset/pdf/Handbook_on_ICMR_Ethical_Guidelines.pdf [Last accessed October, 2021].
6. Kurpad SS. Ethics in psychosocial interventions. Indian J Psychiatry. 2018;60(Suppl 4):S571-S574.
7. Isaac R. Ethics in the practice of clinical psychology. Indian J Medical Ethics. 2009;6(2):69-74.

8. Strous RD. Psychiatry during the Nazi era: ethical lessons for the modern professional. Ann Gen Psychiatry. 2007;6:8.
9. Bracken-Roche D, Racine E. The vulnerability of psychiatric research participants: Why this research ethics concept needs to be revisited? Can J Psychiatry. 2016;6(1):335-9.
10. World Health Organization. (1992). The ICD-10 classification of mental and behavioral disorders, clinical descriptions and diagnostic guidelines. [Online] Available from: https://apps.who.int/iris/handle/10665/37958 [Last accessed October, 2021].
11. American Psychiatric Association. Diagnostic and Statistical Manual of Mental Disorders, Fifth Edition. Arlington (VA); American Psychiatric Association; 2013.
12. World Health Organization (2018). International classification of diseases for morbidity and mortality statistics (11th revision). [Online] Available from: https://icd.who.int/browse11/l-m/en [Last accessed October, 2021].
13. Sheehan DV, Lecrubier Y, Sheehan KH, Amorim P, Janavs J, Weiller E, et al. The Mini-International Neuropsychiatric Interview (M.I.N.I.): the development and validation of a structured diagnostic psychiatric interview for DSM-IV and ICD-10. J Clin Psychiatry. 1998;59 Suppl 20:22-33.
14. World Health Organization. Division of Mental Health. (1994). Schedules for Clinical Assessment in Neuropsychiatry (SCAN). [Online] Available from: https://apps.who.int/iris/handle/10665/40356 [Last accessed October, 2021].
15. World Health Organization (1997). Composite International Diagnostic Interview. Version 2.1. [Online] Available from: https://pubs.niaaa.nih.gov/publications/assessingalcohol/InstrumentPDFs/20_CIDI.pdf [Last accessed October, 2021].
16. Pull CB, Cloos JM, Pull-Erpelding MC. Clinical assessment instruments in psychiatry. In: Maj M, Gaebel W, López-Ibor JJ, Sartorius N (Eds). Psychiatric Diagnosis and Classification. World Psychiatric Association: John Wiley and Sons; 2002. pp. 177-217.
17. Pickersgill MD. Debating DSM5: diagnosis and sociology of critique. J Medical Ethics. 2014;40:521-5.
18. The Mental Healthcare Act. Ministry of law and Justice. The Gazette of India; 2017.
19. The Rights of Persons with Disability Act, 2016. Ministry of Law and Justice. The Gazette of India; 2016.
20. Ali F, Gajera G, Gowda GS, Srinivasa P, Gowda M. Consent in current psychiatric practice and research: an Indian perspective. Indian J Psychiatry. 2019;61(Suppl 4):S667-75.
21. Dubois J, Bante H, Hadley WB. Ethics in psychiatric research: A review of 25 years of NIH funded empirical research projects. AJOB Prim Res. 2011;2(4):5-17.
22. Indian Council of Medical Research (2017). National Ethical Guidelines for Biomedical Research Involving Children. [Online] Available form: https://thsti.res.in/pdf/National_Ethical_Guidelines_for_BioMedical_Research_Involving_Children.pdf [Last accessed October, 2021].
23. United Nations. Convention on the Rights of Persons with Disabilities. Geneva: United Nations Publications; 2006.
24. Mental Health and Human Rights. Annual report of the United Nations High Commissioner for Human Rights. United Nations General Assembly; 2017.
25. Duffy RM, Kelly BD. Concordance of the Indian mental healthcare act 2017 with the World Health Organization's checklist on mental health legislation. Int J Ment Health Syst. 2017;11(1):1-24.
26. World Health Organization (2005). WHO resource book on mental health, human rights and legislation. [Online] Available from: https://ec.europa.eu/health/sites/default/files/mental_health/docs/who_resource_book_en.pdf [Last accessed October, 2021].
27. Philip S, Rangarajan SK, Moirangthem S, Kumar CN, Gowda MR, Gowda GS, et al. Advance directives and nominated representatives: a critique. Indian J Psychiatry. 2019;61(Suppl 4):S680.
28. New Drugs and Clinical Trials Rules. The Gazette of India, Ministry of Health and Family Welfare, Extraordinary, 19 March 2019, Part II, section 3, subsection (i). Supplementary schedule 3, 2 (g), pp. 209-10.
29. George DE, Dholakia S, Tharyan P. Assessing the capacity of psychiatric inpatients and their key relatives to consent to participate in randomised controlled trials. Indian J Med Ethics. 2018;3(2):125-33.
30. Namboodiri V. Capacity for mental health care decisions under the Mental Health Care Act. Indian J Psychiatry. 2019;61(Suppl 4):S676-79.
31. Chen DT, Miller FG, Rosenstein DL. Enrolling decisionally impaired adults in clinical research. Med Care. 2002;40(9 Suppl):V20-9.
32. Helmchen H, Müller-Oerlinghausen B. The inherent paradox of clinical trials in psychiatry. J Med Ethics. 1975;1(4):168-73.
33. DuVal G. Ethics in psychiatric research. Study design issues. Can J Psychiatry. 2004;49(1):55-9.
34. Tharyan P. Ethics in psychiatric research. Indian Journal of Psychiatry. Clinical Practice Guidelines; 2009.
35. World Medical Association (2018). WMA Declaration of Helsinki-Ethical principles for medical research involving human subjects. [Online] Available from: https://www.wma.net/policies-post/wma-declaration-of-helsinki-ethical-principles-for-medical-research-involving-human-subjects/ [Last accessed October, 2021].
36. Skierka AS, Michels KB. Ethical principles and placebo-controlled trials–interpretation and implementation of the Declaration of Helsinki's placebo paragraph in medical research. BMC Medical Ethics. 2018;19(1):1-2.
37. Nugent AC, Miller FG, Helene ID, Zarate CA. The ethics of clinical trials in severe mood disorders. Bioethics. 2017;31(6):443-53.
38. Prasad V, Cifu AS. The necessity of sham controls. Am J Med. 2019;132(2):e29-e30.
39. Miller FG, Kaptchuk TJ. Sham procedures and the ethics of clinical trials. Journal of the Royal Society of Medicine. 2004;97(12):576-8.
40. Enck P, Zipfel S. Placebo effects in psychotherapy: a framework. Front Psychiatry. 2019;10:456.
41. Cunningham JA, Kypri K, McCambridge J. Exploratory randomized controlled trial evaluating the impact of a waiting list control design. BMC Med Res Methodol. 2013;13:150.
42. Berk M, Parker G. The elephant on the couch: side effects of psychotherapy. Aust N Z J Psychiatry. 2009;43(9):787-94.
43. Czaja SJ, Schulz R, Belle SH, Burgio LD, Armstrong N, Gitlin LN, et al. Data and safety monitoring on social behavioral intervention trials: the REACH II experience. Clinical Trials. 2006;3(2):107-18.
44. George DE, Dholakia SA, Tharyan PR. Participation in randomised controlled trials: perspectives of psychiatric

patients and key relatives. Indian journal of medical ethics. 2018;3(1):9-15.
45. Council for International Organizations of Medical Sciences (CIOMS) in collaboration with the World Health Organization (WHO) (2016). International Ethical Guidelines for health related research involving humans. [Online] Available from: https://cioms.ch/wp-content/uploads/2017/01/WEB-CIOMS-EthicalGuidelines.pdf [Last accessed October, 2021].
46. Kurpad SS. High risk sexual behavior—ethical implications, considerations, concerns and dilemmas. In: Cooper DB (Ed). Ethics in Mental Health-Substance Use. Oxford/New York: Routledge; 2017.
47. Avasthi A, Ghosh A, Sarkar S, Grover S. Ethics in medical research: General principles with special reference to psychiatric research. Indian J Psychiatry. 2013;55(1):86-91.
48. Gearing RE, Mian IA, Barber J, Icklowicz A. A methodology for conducting retrospective chart review research in child and adolescent psychiatry. J Can Acad Child Adolesc Psychiatry. 2006;15(3):126-34.
49. Choudhury S, Ghosh A. Ethical considerations of mental health research amidst COVID-19 pandemic: Mitigating the challenges. Indian J Psychol Med. 2020;42(4):379-81.
50. Cosgrove V, Gliddon E, Berk L, Grimm D, Lauder S, Dodd S, et al. Online ethics: where will the interface of mental health and the internet lead us? Int J Bipolar Disord. 2017;5(1):1-9.
51. Buchanan EA, Zimmer M. Internet Research Ethics. The Stanford Encyclopedia of Philosophy (Summer 2021 Edition). [Online] Available from: https://plato.stanford.edu/cgi-bin/encyclopedia/archinfo.cgi?entry=ethics-internet-research [Last accessed October, 2021].
52. Franzke AS, Bechmann A, Zimmer M, Ess CM; the Association of Internet Researchers. (2019). Internet Research: Ethical Guidelines 3.0. [Online] Available from: https://aoir.org/reports/ethics3.pdf [Last accessed October, 2021].
53. World Health Organization (2010). Research ethics in international epidemic response. [Online] Available from: https://apps.who.int/iris/handle/10665/70739 [Last accessed October, 2021].
54. World Health Organization (2015). Ethics in epidemics, emergencies and disasters: research, surveillance and patient care. Training manual. [Online] Available from: https://www.who.int/publications/i/item/ethics-in-epidemics-emergencies-and-disasters-research-surveillance-and-patient-care-training-manual [Last accessed October, 2021].
55. Taquet M, Luciano S, Geddes JR, Harrison PJ. Bidirectional associations between COVID-19 and psychiatric disorder: retrospective cohort studies of 62 354 COVID-19 cases in the USA. Lancet Psychiatry. 2021;8(2):130-40.
56. Holmes EA, O'Connor RC, Perry VH, Tracey I, Wessely S, Arseneault L, et al. Multidisciplinary research priorities for the COVID-19 pandemic: a call for action for mental health science. Lancet Psychiatry. 2020;7(6):547-60.
57. Glasziou PP, Sanders S, Hoffmann T. Waste in COVID-19 research. BMJ. 2020;369:m1847.
58. Altman DG. The scandal of poor medical research. BMJ. 1994;308(6924):283-4.
59. Kumar M, Sandhu H, Roshan R. Indian Council of Medical Research's International Collaboration & Partnerships; Health Ministry's Screening Committee: Facts, figures & procedures. Indian J Med Res. 2020;151(6):550-3.
60. Fulford KW, Howse K. Ethics of research with psychiatric patients: principles, problems and the primary responsibilities of researchers. J Med Ethics. 1993;19(2):85-91.
61. Miller FG, Rosenstein DL, DeRenzo EG. Professional integrity in clinical research. JAMA. 1998;280:1449-54.
62. Executive of the Faculty of Academic Psychiatry of the Royal College of Psychiatrists. Ethics of Psychiatric Research. Position Statement PS02. Royal College of Psychiatry, UK. 2011. [online] Available from: https://www.rcpsych.ac.uk/docs/default-source/members/faculties/academic-psychiatry/academic-research-ethics-of-psychiatric-research.pdf?sfvrsn=cc46dd6_2 [Last accessed January, 2021].

CHAPTER 6

Ethics of International Collaboration in Biomedical and Health Research: An Indian Perspective

Mukesh Kumar

ABSTRACT

Various international partnerships in research continue to grow, and these have evolved with time from input-driven to output-driven research. We are no longer in a position to generate all the know-how in one single research laboratory from the initial research to the final product. For this reason, we are turning more and more to teamwork in partnership with academic (research institutes, universities, medical colleges, and hospitals) and industrial entities (established players and start-ups) globally. There is a growing realization that national, regional, and global partnerships might expedite the whole process of finding solutions for various health and other societal challenges. Necessary byelaws, guidelines, rules, regulations, and any issues related to culture, religion, politics, etc., of all countries involved in joint research projects should be respected by researchers from all collaborating countries. This would include intellectual property (IP) rights, transfer of biological materials (human, animal, plant or microbial), issues related to data transfer, security/sensitivity, etc. With respect to the Indian scenario, any research requiring transfer of biological materials abroad should have the duly filled and signed material transfer agreement (MTA) document with justification for the purpose and information about postanalysis handling, disposal, and safety during sample transfer, etc. The international collaborative research in India, with or without foreign funds, should be peer reviewed and guided by the respective Ethics Committee (EC). Projects in biomedical research involving foreign assistance and/or collaboration are required to be submitted to the Health Ministry's Screening Committee (HMSC) for review and decision before initiation.

INTRODUCTION

International collaboration in biomedical and health research is becoming increasingly relevant to reap the benefits of the latest newer advances in Science and Technology (S&T) for better application to public health in any country. There is a strong need to promote a culture of innovation and research to target-oriented, specific product development in health sciences, such as cost-effective and robust vaccines and low-cost medicines for the common man, either independently or through appropriate international partners. India has been contributing to the development of various global strategies and plans in this respect.

India has an advantage in International Cooperation (IC) because of its vast domestic market, huge educated/skilled workforce, progressive scientific community, growing economy, state-of-the-art facilities, cost-effective infrastructure, and, more importantly, self-reliance in many sectors. India has undertaken many steps in shaping the future of its next generation through international collaborations by facilitating the development of appropriate technologies. The motto is to generate knowledge and share its fruits globally for a win–win situation. There is also a great interest in establishing public–private partnerships involving international partners.

Today, the benefits of IC are flowing back to the society in the form of trained manpower in big or small academic institutions as well as in the biotechnology industry. In the recent past, India has opened several new channels of IC based on mutual respect and trust. We are no longer in a position to generate all the know-how in one single academic research institution or laboratory. This has created the need for doing quality research with the involvement of international stakeholders.

The rationale of global joint efforts has its roots in common issues and priorities to tackle shared problems, developing networks as well as providing timely and relevant solutions. IC is better today than at any time in the past. We need to invest more time, money, and energy in working together to deal with great challenges and bring the benefits of science from bench to bedside and from laboratory to land, thereby translating it from discovery science to solution and application science.

This could result in building the capacity of academic institutes, thorough strengthening of trained manpower, infrastructure, and technology development. Generally, biomedical research/public health and health research are prominently covered in almost all bilateral Memorandum of Understandings (MoUs) in S&T. Additionally, there are some specific instruments signed by the Ministry of Health and Family Welfare (MoHFW) with other countries, as well as some are signed by the Indian Council of Medical Research (ICMR) directly with its counterpart international organizations/institutions. Currently, there are nearly two dozen bilateral MoUs/Letters of Intent (LoIs)/Joint Statements involving ICMR with various international organizations/institutions (www.icmr.nic.in).[1] Many more such arrangements are either under negotiation or in the approval process.

The purposes of these MoUs/instruments are as follows:
- Joint execution of scientific projects, including support in the procurement of scientific equipment
- Exchange of scientists/researchers for training under the approved projects
- Exchange of scientific information
- Organization of joint scientific meetings, seminars, workshops, symposia, and conferences in common areas of cooperation

MODES OF INTERNATIONAL COLLABORATION

With increase in globalization, international collaboration has also increased. Presently, other than data exchange, seminars, workshops, and collaborative joint research projects, there are several new modes of collaboration, such as building of networks, fellowships, and consortia for boosting academic research careers through the exchange of scientists as well as mobility from one country to another. Scientific democracy is knowledge economy or co-evolution of science and society/democracy in this era of competitiveness, through innovations in S&T. Scientists have shown great promise for S&T cooperation with the developing countries. Such coordinated and collective efforts are likely to bring direct benefits to the people.

Many countries are promoting access and participation in major international facilities, such as Facility for Antiproton and Ion Research (FAIR) in Germany, European Synchrotron Radiation Facility (ESRF) and European Organization for Nuclear Research (CERN) in France, and the High Energy Accelerator Research Organization (KEK) and Super Photon ring-8 GeV (SPring-8) in Japan. Many Centers of Excellence in Science have come up in the recent past. India is attracting senior scientists living abroad through dedicated programs and schemes to provide exposure to young researchers, and international fellowships are being offered by various S&T departments and organizations.

The above forms of collaborations help in imparting training by organizing thematic/summer schools to decide on research priorities that are important for each of the partnering countries. Such efforts in IC are required these days for interactive dissemination of knowledge and information by working on a common plank with other departments/agencies to coordinate and draw maximum benefits. There are several international institutions and agencies that have existing collaborative ties with India in biomedical research, especially for innovations for tackling epidemic preparedness, such as the recent epidemics and the COVID-19 pandemic, which may result in a syndemic.

New Growth Models of International Cooperation

In the recent past, India has built up expertise in upgrading the skills of scientists and researchers of academic institutions in various fields and at different places. There have been many attempts to help other countries in South-East Asia Region and SAARC to address various issues in health research, such as the Regional Enabler for South-East Asia Research Collaboration for Health (RESEARCH). This platform was launched in 2019 to combat dangerous pathogens/emerging and re-emerging diseases in the South-East Asian countries.

The efforts will be made to include more countries in the network. This expertise is being shared with neighboring developing countries for the transfer of technology and training in cutting-edge as well as classical scientific disciplines. Such multidisciplinary cooperation is likely to bring maximum benefits and increase cost-effective productivity. Another example is the formalization of the India–Africa partnership by establishing an India–Africa Health Sciences Platform (IAHSP). This is a partnership of two regions for optimal use of resources in health sciences. Some other important examples are the Vaccine Action Program (VAP) with USA, the Coalition for Epidemic Preparedness Innovations (CEPI) with headquarters in Norway and bi-national centers under intergovernmental arrangements with France (IFCPAR/CEFIPRA), USA (IUSSTF), and Germany (IGSTC).

There is a need for open and constructive dialogues on a continuous basis, development of strategic partnership in key sectors with co-investment of resources, joint co-ownership of IP, and co-generation of such results for capacity strengthening by developing common technological platforms. Our basic fundamental of inclusive growth and sustainable development should work more and more to ensure drawing maximum from minimum, thus making the "impossible" into a "possible" outcome.

COLLABORATIVE RESEARCH IN HEALTH SCIENCES

Research in health sciences has achieved greater height in the recent past. The international collaboration has become a necessity for both developing and developed world. The scope of IC and collaboration has assumed such proportions as to have exploitative connotations with commercial and human dimensions. The collaboration in health research is in accordance with requirement of mankind and is undertaken through experimentation on the population of different regions and countries. In view of fast globalization, economic competition, and need to protect IP, it is necessary to find cost-effective approaches in international collaboration to boost scientific productivity and technology development. Similar experience is applicable even when there is no collaboration between the countries; however, research is undertaken with financial assistance from a funder as sponsor (public or private or philanthropic). The collaboration may involve implementation of multiple components of the research or even a single component, such as laboratory testing.[2]

There are formal bilateral/multilateral collaborative S&T arrangements between research organizations of the Government of India (GOI) and similar bodies of several other countries, which are mainly coordinated by the Department of Science & Technology (DST), Department of Biotechnology (DBT) and Council of Scientific and Industrial Research (CSIR), etc. ICMR is represented in some of them for components related to health sciences.

ROLE AND COMPOSITION OF HEALTH MINISTRY'S SCREENING COMMITTEE

The HMSC is an inter-ministerial committee constituted by the MoHFW, GOI, in the early 1980s. All biomedical research involving foreign assistance and/or collaboration should necessarily be submitted to the HMSC for review and approval before initiation (details can be accessed at https://main.icmr.nic.in/content/guidelines), whether financed (partly/completely) or not financed. However, as per DST OM No. DST/INT/HLC/2006 dated 14/8/2006, "after having satisfied at the level of Secretary of concerned Ministry or Department that no security/sensitivity aspects are involved, they may give clearance". Since the beginning of 2020, the HMSC meets six times in a year on alternate months. Indian researchers willing to have foreign collaboration and/or assistance in health sciences can upload their projects online through ICMR/Department of Health Research (DHR) portal for HMSC. ICMR/DHR is in process of further simplifying the procedures regarding HMSC clearance of collaborative research projects. Recently, it has been decided that the DBT will be the nodal department for an online integrated portal called BioRRAP (Biological Research Regulatory Approval Portal), which will be linked with HMSC portal also for necessary, centralized information and regulatory mechanism on international projects.

Composition of HMSC

The ICMR/DHR functions as the technical arm for HMSC and conducts technical evaluation of the international research projects. The International Health Division (IHD) in ICMR Headquarters (Hqrs.) is the Secretariat for HMSC on behalf of DHR and organizes the meetings for placement of collaborative research projects before this committee. The international collaborative health research projects are scientifically reviewed by the Scientific Divisions at ICMR Hqrs., New Delhi, and experts in the fields.

The current composition of the HMSC consists of Secretary, DHR, MoHFW, GOI, who serves as the Chairman, and the members include nominees of Secretary, Health & FW; Addl. Secretary & Director General, NACO; Secretary, AYUSH; Director General of Health Services; Joint Secretary, Department of Health Research; Director General of Armed Forces and Medical Services (DGAFMS); Joint Secretary-Family Planning or Deputy Commissioner-Family Planning; Representative from Ministry of External Affairs (MEA)—Coordination Division; Department of Economic Affairs (DEA); Department of Biotechnology (DBT); Department of Science and Technology (DST); and Head, International Health Division (IHD), ICMR as the Member Secretary on behalf of DHR.

ETHICS OF INTERNATIONAL COLLABORATION

Ethics is an important component in biomedical and health research projects. The responsibility of ECs is to scrutinize the scientific and ethical aspects of the collaborative research proposals undertaken in the implementing country and acts as the conscience keepers of the society.

While the ethical reviews and approvals are subject to the national regulatory framework in each country, the international collaborations attract appropriate considerations for the general ethical principles. Although these principles are common, the specific principles recommended in the Indian context may vary from one country to another because of differences in cultural and social aspects. The review conduct and monitoring of international collaborative research in India should be guided by the respective ECs, which are functioning as prescribed by the ICMR through its National Ethical Guidelines for Biomedical and Health Research involving human participants, 2017, which has now been included in the New Drugs and Clinical Trials (NDCT) Rules, 2019,[3] making its compliance mandatory in the country. From September, 2019, the DHR has set up a National Ethics Committees Registration Portal (www.naitik.gov.in) for all ECs reviewing academic, biomedical, and health research proposals.[4] Each site investigator is responsible for approval of the proposal from the respective EC before consideration for HMSC's approval. Research proposals involving clinical trials should also be registered with the Clinical Trials Registry-India (CTRI).

International Guidelines

The EC approval is an integral part of any grant applications and most research institutes/organizations have full-fledged ECs. According to national guidelines and related international guidelines, EC should be an independent body constituted of medical/nonmedical, scientific, and nonscientific members, responsible for ensuring the protection of the rights, safety, and well-being of human participants in research. Among other things, EC reviews, approves, and conducts continuing review of research/trial protocols and their amendments and how informed consent of the trial participants is administered and documented.

The research proposals need to follow the ethical guidelines/regulations of their respective countries. The Council for International Organizations of Medical Sciences (CIOMS) released "International Ethical Guidelines for Health-Related Research involving human subjects (2016), which provides a framework for research having international collaboration,[5] wherein it is stated that research ECs and health authorities have a moral obligation to ensure that all research is carried out in ways that uphold human rights, protect and respect study participants and the communities in which the research is conducted." In addition, the research proposals need to declare that good clinical and laboratory practices will be followed and the research study will be conducted in accordance with the Helsinki Declaration on "ethical principles for medical research involving human subjects (https://www.wma.net/policies-post/wma-declaration-of-helsinki-ethical-principles-for-medical-research-involving-human-subjects/)."

In 2018, a Global Code of Conduct (GCC) for research in resource-poor settings has been brought out by TRUST consortium with funding from European Commission, which is made mandatory for EU funded projects to follow while conducting collaborative research with low- and middle-income countries (LMICs) to improve adherence to high ethical standards in scientific research around the world.[6] GCC is currently being followed in 40 countries with emphasis on four principles—respect, fairness, care, and honesty and aims to stop the export of unethical research practices or "ethics dumping" to resource-poor settings to achieve fair partnerships in research. This has been translated into multiple languages including Hindi.

ROLE OF ETHICS COMMITTEES

The ECs should strictly review/scrutinize proposals taking into account various ethical aspects of the proposal and should ensure that a scientific evaluation has been completed before ethics review is taken up. It is crucial to follow the ethical guidelines as it helps to promote the aims of research and the ethos that are essential for collaborative study. Where the research involves international collaboration between researchers from advanced and less advanced countries, it should assess its acceptability to local customs, traditions, and heritage to avoid risk of exploitation, which may lead to inequalities, e.g., financial, access to resources, etc., between the project collaborators. Often, the knowledge derived from the research does not benefit the target population and/or the host organization. Sometimes, study designs are used where the control or placebo group receives no treatment/care or disease screening, even if an optimal standard of care/screening is available (https://link.springer.com/chapter/10.1007/978-3-319-64731-9_5). Such studies should only be allowed if the control or placebo patients are not subjected to harm as a result of taking part in the research study. The term "ethics dumping" coined by the European Commission aptly describes the unethical practices adopted by developed countries while collaborating with the LMICs and the GCC mentioned above has been specifically developed to prevent such instances. In this regard, the TRUST, EU funded project, has brought out a publication on Ethics Dumping,[7] giving examples of real-time case studies, which describe the different types of unethical practices that have been applied in international collaborations. Hence, it is important for ECs of all participating countries to see overall that risks and benefits are equitably distributed and continuously monitored. Prior to initiating the research work, the ECs should assess the risks and benefits to individuals participating in research. The Informed Consent Document (ICD) submitted by the investigator should describe in simple language, the study procedures, risks, and benefits, and ensure that there is an opportunity and capacity in the participant to understand and decide whether to participate or refuse without having been subjected to any undue influence. Even if there is a global template for informed consent, a site-specific ICD to suit the local cultural sensitivities should be prepared by the researcher and approved by the local ECs, which should be acceptable to the international collaborator.

CONCERNS ON ETHICAL ISSUES AND HMSC SUBMISSION

Any international collaborative research study to be conducted in India necessitates that all regulatory requirements are to be followed and complied with. The magnitude and severity of the health-related problems are different in different countries; capacity building to address ethical issues in collaborative research is required to be promoted first. Procedures should be followed and implemented so that participating countries and communities can practice and implement meaningful self-determination in healthcare upliftment while ensuring scientific and ethical conduct of research. For Indian collaborative research, the following key points should be considered:

- The Indian participating researchers should function as equal partners with the foreign collaborators and sponsors. Equality means equal ownership of data, equal rights to analyze, disseminate, and publish the data, and equal sharing of IP rights as required.
- There must be bilateral/multilateral free flow of knowledge and capacity. Assignees based on their contribution should be credited for the IP rights.

- Careful consideration should be given to respect the dignity, safety/security, and welfare of the participants particularly when the social contexts of the proposed research can create difficult situation for them by exploitation and/or increase their vulnerability to harm. The corrective initiatives should be taken to overcome such matters with prior approval taken from concerned EC.
- The informed consent is required to be taken from each and every adult participant in the study. In case of a child or a cognitively impaired participant or any other vulnerable participant as specified in the National Ethical Guidelines, her/his assent, as may be applicable should be obtained along with the consent of the parent or the legally authorized/acceptable representative (LAR).
- As different kinds of research have their own particular scientific need and specific ethical challenges, the selection of study participants should be justified in accordance with science and ethics. By and large, early clinical phases of research, particularly of drugs, vaccines, tools, and devices, should be conducted in populations that are less vulnerable to harm or exploitation.
- The nature, magnitude, and probability of all foreseeable loss resulting from participation in a collaborative research should be specified in the research protocol and explained fully to the participants at the beginning.
- All participants in the research should have access to the best possible or optimal care available in the country. Moreover, other modalities including provision for compensation for injury and/or death (adverse events/serious adverse events) following the research, and subsequent referral for psychosocial/medical aid and legal support if required, need to be explained. The EC should ensure and monitor whether appropriate clinical care, compensation, and other supports, as applicable, are provided to the participants.
- The research protocol should outline the benefits that persons/communities participating in such research should experience. Care should be taken to ensure that these are presented in a way that do not unduly influence the freedom of choice in their participation. Any loss or benefit should be equally distributed among the collaborating institutions and sponsor/agencies.
- There should be an appropriate mechanism for communication between the ECs of all the participating centers and each of the centers should provide EC clearance. In case of any conflict, the decision of the EC in the host country shall prevail and will be considered as final.

Guidelines and Regulations

Guidelines, rules, regulations, and local laws as well as any form of cultural, religious, regional, social/tribal, political, cast, and creed sensitivities of all countries participating in collaborative research projects should be respected, especially by researchers from the research implementing country and the sponsor country. The national security is of prime importance without compromising country's integrity. These could be with reference to IP rights, exchange of biological materials (human, animal, plant or microbial), data transfer, its protection as well as its safety/security issues. The study cannot be a data capturing platform only with no contribution to the enhancement of knowledge base of partners.

- In this context, it is essential for researchers to follow the GOI notification on "Exchange of Human Biological Material for Biomedical Research" issued on November 19, 1997, vide F.No.L.19015/53/97-IH(Pt.), by MoHFW, GOI (can be accessed at http://www.icmr.nic.in/min.htm). Any research involving import or export of biological specimen to the collaborating institution(s) outside India must submit the duly filled and signed MTA document with justification for the purpose of transfer and also mention about post-analysis handling and disposal. Export of samples for quality control measure must not exceed the recommended limit. Research projects requiring transfer of biological material and quantity beyond the recommended limit for quality assurance and quality control purposes may be considered by the EC on a case-to-case basis because its recommendations will guide HMSC to make the final decision.
- Collaborators should obtain appropriate regulatory clearances as prevalent in the country, such as Environmental Protection Act 1986; The Biological Diversity Act 2002; Drugs and Cosmetics Act 1940/Rules 1945 and its recent amendment; the NDCT Rules, 2019,[3] etc., and obtain EC approval from all participating centers before the initiation of the study.
- The Indian participating center(s) must have all regulatory approvals as required for receiving foreign funds for research under Foreign Contribution (Regulation) Act (FCRA), 2010 and its Amendment Bill, 2020.[8]
- It is necessary to abide by the Directorate General of Foreign Trade (DGFT) notification "No. 19/2015-2020 dated August 4, 2016, related to transfer of human biological material for commercial purposes: to facilitate import/export of human biological samples for commercial purposes" by the Indian Clinical Research Organizations (CRO'S)/Diagnostic Laboratories. Amendment Schedule-1 (Import Policy) and Schedule-2 (Export Policy) of ITC (HS), 2012, DGFT notification are available on ICMR and DGFT websites.[9]
- Approval of Drugs Controller General of India (DCGI) is required in case of global clinical trials.
- Registration with CTRI is mandatory and should be obtained before the study has started recruiting participants (CTRI was launched by ICMR in 2007; approximately 32,470 trials/research have been registered till March 31, 2021).

- Nongovernmental organizations are to be empaneled with NITI Aayog (NGO Darpan Portal) and should also submit certain other requisite documents as prescribed.
- Requisite clearances are needed if study involves working with radiotagged material and recombinant DNA/genetic engineering work [issued by BARC and DBT (RCGM), respectively].
- Guidelines are to be followed on foreign engagement on Bio-safety/Bio-security matters (dated December, 2015) prepared and issued by Division of Disarmament & International Security Affairs (D&ISA), MEA (duly approved by GOI), for compliance in order to protect national security [Weapons of Mass Destruction Act, 2005 and overall framework of Biological and Toxin Weapons Convention (BTWC)][10,11].
- The Nagoya Protocol on Access and Benefit Sharing (ABS), a new international treaty adopted under the auspices of the Convention on Biological Diversity (CBD) in Nagoya, Japan in 2010, which aims at fair and equitable sharing of benefits arising from the utilization of genetic resources, should also be followed.

SOME PRACTICAL ILLUSTRATIONS ON WORKING OF EC

A few recurring issues have been noticed in the projects submitted and reviewed by HMSC (lists of up-to-date projects approved by HMSC in last more than 21 years, from January 2000, onward are available on the ICMR website). For instance, the issues recorded below were observed when 136 proposals involving foreign collaboration and/or assistance approved by HMSC from June 1 to December 31, 2018, were considered for analysis.[12] Suggestions based on these project reviews have also been compiled, which will be useful for the investigators and the ECs for consideration in future **(Table 1)**.

Some Examples of Unethical Practices Observed in International Collaborations

- Studies conducted without HMSC or required necessary approvals.
  - Studies not relevant to local population (BA/BE studies performed for drugs that are not marketed locally).
  - Following double standards in ethical requirements (use of placebo in developing countries when optimal standard care is available).
- Failure to submit periodic progress and final reports to regulators and funders.
- Extension of the project's duration on request by the sponsors, without approval.
- Data published in international journals without necessary approval, sharing of only de-identified or anonymized data for statistical or other purposes needs to be considered, while
  - Ensuring that proper data sharing agreement has been drawn up. Each site investigator is responsible for only her/his site-specific data and its accessibility.
  - Lack of provision of compensation or insurance cover for the participants for injuries incurred during the research period.
  - Under the plea that the research is an educational activity, fellowship or scholarship, some ECs approve the research, allowing it to escape regulatory approval route.

TABLE 1: Issues observed in projects submitted for HMSC review and suggestions for the same.

Issues	Suggestions
About 28% of EC letters did not mention the composition of the committees.	All EC approval letters submitted to the funding agencies should mention the composition of ECs.
Only 50% of EC approval letters submitted by Principal Investigators (PIs) indicated that all the necessary documents were received and reviewed by the EC.	The minutes of the EC and the approval letters should list the documents with version numbers that were considered and approved.
Only 65% of EC approval letters had mentioned validity period of EC clearance in their letters.	Approval by the EC should be for the project duration. If there is delay in initiating the project, fresh approval or extension should be sought from the EC. It is necessary to indicate the validity period of the EC approval, since many times the final approval for initiation of the project comes after the EC-approved time frame. However, even then, instead of asking for fresh approval or extension of approval for the validity period from the EC, the PIs initiate the study. Such instances are treated as noncompliance to guidelines.
ECs ask for additional documents, such as letters from CTRI, DCGI, or even an MoU before initiation of the study and provide additional comments in the interest of science.	The required documents should be submitted and the comments should be complied with by the PIs. There are instances where one EC gives approval for many sites. It is desirable to have a specified format for submission of papers to ECs and provide them with a checklist for some kind of uniformity. In this context, the draft guidelines of ICMR for multicentric studies and use of its Common Submission Forms should be followed.[13,14]

(HMSC: Health Ministry's Screening Committee; EC: Ethics Committee; MoU: memorandum of understanding; CTRI: Clinical Trials Registry–India; DCGI: Drugs Controller General of India)

- Transfer of biological samples without approval and without MTA, when transfer is not an integral part of a collaborative research project.
  - Results from research studies using biological samples from India are published in scientific journals without an Indian collaborator or author.
  - Lack of research component in studies with the sole aim of transfer of biological samples.
  - ECs are giving waiver from ethical angle for projects that involve human participants, including transfer of biological materials and data.
  - Lack of seriousness in following safety guidelines during transfer of hazardous samples.
  - The original project approved by HMSC or equivalent committee lacks mention of transfer of samples at any stage, but it is later proposed or considered to transfer biological samples. If so, permissible percentage of samples will be allowed to be transferred, provided proper justification for reconsideration and reversal of the previous decision is provided in advance to the approving authorities.
  - The original project approved by HMSC or equivalent committee had indication for transfer of X number of samples to single foreign laboratory, whereas the principal investigator (PI) of the project subsequently transfers X+ samples to many laboratories outside the country.
  - There is no mention of long-term storage of samples in the study, but later on the PI decides to do so (patient/participant information sheet and consent form should have clearly mentioned the plans for long-term storage, the investigations, and the type of analysis to be done using the participants' biological samples).
  - Many times, extension of the study duration is sought only with the aim of transferring stored samples.

CONCLUSION

There is a great interest among researchers for developing partnerships with foreign researchers in biomedical research. ICMR is actively involved in the co-funding and coordinating these partnership programs with many international organizations and agencies. Various MoUs/DoI/MoI of ICMR with international counterpart agencies bring together researchers and resources toward progression through shared research and innovation agenda. Growing collaborations during recent years are reflected through an increasing number of internationally funded/technically coordinated research projects in health research. However, for any meaningful, beneficial, and nonexploitative collaborative research study to be undertaken in India, the relevant ethical and regulatory requirements should be fulfilled, respected, and strictly complied with.

REFERENCES

1. Indian Council of Medical Research. ICMR Guidelines for International Collaboration/Research Projects in Health Research; MoUs& HMSC Procedure. [online] Available from: https://main.icmr.nic.in/content/guidelines [Last accessed October, 2021].
2. Indian Council of Medical Research (2017). National Ethical Guidelines for biomedical and health research involving human participants. [online] Available from: https://main.icmr.nic.in/sites/default/files/guidelines/ICMR_Ethical_Guidelines_2017.pdf.
3. Central Drugs Standard Control Organisation. New Drugs and Clinical Trials Rules, 2019. [online] Available from: https://cdsco.gov.in/opencms/export/sites/CDSCO_WEB/Pdf-documents/NewDrugs_CTRules_2019.pdf [Last accessed October, 2021].
4. Department of Health Research. National Ethics Committee Registry for Biomedical and Health Research (NECRBHR), 2019. [online] Available from: https://dhr.gov.in/national-ethics-committee-registry-biomedical-and-health-research-necrbhr [Last accessed October, 2021].
5. Council for International Organizations of Medical Sciences (2016). International ethical guidelines for health-related research involving humans. [online] Available from: https://cioms.ch/publications/product/international-ethical-guidelines-for-health-related-research-involving-humans [Last accessed October, 2021].
6. TRUST. Global Code of Conduct for Research in Resource-Poor Settings, 2018. [online] Available from: https://www.globalcodeofconduct.org/ [Last accessed October, 2021].
7. Schroeder D, Cook J, Hirsch F, Fenet S, Muthuswamy V (Eds). Ethics Dumping: Case Studies from North-South Research Collaborations. Switzerland: Springer; 2018.
8. Foreign Contribution (Regulation) Amendment Bill (FCRA), 2010/2020. [online] Available from: https://fcraonline.nic.in/home/PDF_Doc/fc_amend_07102020_1.pdf [Last accessed October, 2021].
9. Directorate General of Foreign Trade, Rules. [online] Available from: https://www.dgft.gov.in/CP/?opt=fdt-rules [Last accessed October, 2021].
10. Ministry of External Affairs, Government of India. The Weapons of Mass Destruction and their Delivery Systems (Prohibition of Unlawful Activities) Act. Act I.D: 200521. [Internet} New Delhi: Gazette of India; 2005. Available from: https://www.indiacode.nic.in/handle/123456789/2017?view_type=search&sam_handle=123456789/1362.
11. The Nuclear Threat Initiative. Convention on the Prohibition of the Development, Production and Stockpiling of Bacteriological (Biological) and Toxin Weapons (BTWC). [Internet]. Washington, DC. Available from: https://www.nti.org/education-center/treaties-and-regimes/convention-prohibition-development-production-and-stockpiling-bacteriological-biological-and-toxin-weapons-btwc/
12. Kumar M, Sandhu H, Roshan R. Indian Council of Medical Research's International Collaboration & Partnerships; Health Ministry's Screening Committee: Facts, figures & procedures. Indian J Med Res. 2020;151(6):550-3.
13. ICMR Common Forms for Ethics Committee Review. [online] Available from: https://main.icmr.nic.in/forms [Last accessed October, 2021].
14. Indian Council of Medical Research (2019). Draft ICMR Guidelines for Common Ethics Review of Multicentre Research. Available from: https://main.icmr.nic.in/sites/default/files/guidelines/Draft_ICMR_Guidelines.pdf [Last accessed October, 2021].

CHAPTER 7

Ethical Issues in Assisted Reproductive Technologies

Puvithra Thanikachalam, Radha Pandiyan, Pandiyan Natarajan

ABSTRACT

Assisted reproductive technology (ART) has become an integral part of infertility treatment. The rapid progress and advancement in this field have evoked concerns regarding the ethical issues related to its practice. Ethics in assisted reproduction is not only about the rights of a single individual, but also extends to the safety and rights of the infertile couple, their embryos and progeny, the donor or the surrogate in case of third-party reproduction, and the community, society, and world at large. Third-party reproduction involves a higher degree of insight and implementation of ethical considerations. This chapter discusses the ethical issues related to ART procedures, the various ethical dilemmas arising from them, and also the present guidelines and regulations pertaining to them. Implementation of guidelines for the practice of ART in India could mitigate the risk of exploitation of all individuals involved including the ART practitioners.

INTRODUCTION

Medical ethics pertains to the physician's responsibilities to patients, healthcare organizations, and society. The practice of any branch of medicine should enable addressing the social and cultural ethos of its community.[1] Universal ethics is more difficult to understand or implement as standards and norms vary globally. Due to the ever-changing norms which apply to ethics, ethical issues related to assisted reproduction need constant understanding and evolution. New technologies in assisted reproduction bring their own ethical concerns adding a dimension that may need considerable deliberation. Infertility is defined as "the inability to conceive after 1 year of regular unprotected intercourse."[2] While population control has been a worldwide concern, the impact of infertility on couples is considerable. Among all couples in the reproductive age group, 15% are infertile and 70% of these couples require some form of assisted reproduction.[2] Infertility is not only a medical problem, but also has social implications requiring physical, mental, spiritual, emotional, financial, and social support.

REPRODUCTION: A FUNDAMENTAL RIGHT

The World Health Organization defines reproductive rights as "the recognition of the basic right of all couples and individuals to decide freely and responsibly the number, spacing and timing of their children and to have the information and means to do so, and the right to attain the highest standard of sexual and reproductive health. They also include the right of all to make decisions concerning reproduction free of discrimination, coercion, and violence." Procreation is the basis for sustenance of any species and reproduction is considered as one of the fundamental rights of every individual.[3] There is a considerable difference in personal preferences when it comes to when to reproduce, how many children to have, the spacing between children, and their choice of contraceptive practice.[1,4]

There has always been a debate on whether infertility treatment should be offered when there is overgrowing population. There are arguments against this stating that the societal burden of overpopulation should not be carried by the infertile couple alone.[5]

ASSISTED REPRODUCTIVE TECHNOLOGIES

Assisted reproductive technologies are defined as "techniques which involve the in vitro manipulation of the oocyte and spermatozoa." In current parlance, even intrauterine insemination (IUI) is sometimes termed ART. The various technologies available for men and women are mentioned in **Table 1**.[6]

Even though the first IVF baby Louise Brown was born on July 25, 1978, by the pioneering efforts of Dr Patrick Steptoe, Sir Robert Edwards, and Ms Purdy, they were not duly recognized until 2010, when Professor Edwards was awarded the Nobel Prize for his contribution. In the early days, the practice of assisted reproduction evoked criticism regarding ethical and religious issues.

TABLE 1: Assisted reproductive techniques (Terminologies adapted from the International Glossary on Infertility and Fertility Care, 2017).

Procedures	Definition
Gamete intrafallopian transfer (GIFT)	An ART procedure in which both gametes (oocytes and spermatozoa) are transferred into a fallopian tube(s)
Zygote intrafallopian transfer (ZIFT)	An ART procedure in which one or more zygotes is transferred into the fallopian tube
In vitro fertilization (IVF)	A sequence of procedures that involves extracorporeal fertilization of gametes
Intracytoplasmic sperm injection (ICSI)	A procedure in which a single spermatozoon is injected into the oocyte cytoplasm
Percutaneous epididymal sperm aspiration (PESA)	A surgical procedure in which a needle is introduced percutaneously into the epididymis with the intention of obtaining spermatozoa
Microsurgical epididymal sperm aspiration (MESA)	A surgical procedure performed with the assistance of an operating microscope to retrieve spermatozoa from the epididymis of men with obstructive azoospermia
Testicular sperm extraction (TESE)	A surgical procedure involving one or more testicular biopsies to obtain spermatozoa for use in IVF and/or ICSI
Microsurgical testicular sperm extraction (micro-TESE)	A surgical procedure using an operating microscope to identify seminiferous tubules that may contain spermatozoa to be extracted for ICSI
Gamete donation and IVF/ICSI	The use of oocytes or spermatozoa from a donor for reproductive purposes or research
Surrogacy	Surrogacy is "an arrangement where a surrogate mother bears and delivers a child for another couple or persons who are the genetic parents of the child"

Professor Dr Subhas Mukherjee, India's first architect of ART, created India's first ART baby and the world's second, Ms Kanupriya (Durga) Agarwal. She was born on October 3, 1978. Due to lack of adequate documentation and absence of tolerance and ignorance of the scientific community, Dr Mukherjee faced condemnation and criticism driving him to commit suicide.

The first officially recognized IVF baby of India was Ms Harsha Chawda. She was born in Mumbai following IVF done by Professor T C Anand Kumar from the Institute for Research in Reproduction (IRR) and Dr Indira Hinduja of the KEM Hospital in the year 1986. This was 8 years after the first actual Indian IVF birth achieved at Kolkata by Professor Subhas Mukherjee. His monumental work and the subsequent tragic story were revealed to the world by Professor Anand Kumar in 1997 who also celebrated the silver jubilee (25th year) of the first official test tube baby in 2003 and felicitated Ms Kanupriya Agarwal.

Assisted Reproduction in Special Groups

Single Individuals and Individuals of Different Sexual Orientations

Although there is no ambiguity in the belief that reproduction is a fundamental right, yet during specific situations such as offering ART to single men and women or those with different sexual orientations, questions do arise. The recent Government of India ART regulation bill, 2020, forbids single men from availing ART services, considering the welfare of the child, whereas ART is available for single women. Indian law also allows single women to adopt a child. This discrimination has received considerable criticism and is considered to interfere with the reproductive autonomy of single men. The National Institute for Health and Clinical Excellence (NICE) guidelines, UK, on Infertility, released in 2004, did not mention about single women or same-sex couples seeking treatment.[7] This social criterion was later addressed in the Human Fertilization and Embryology Act 2008, UK, which replaced the "need for father" with "the need for supportive parenting."[8]

Physically Challenged/Medically Ill Individuals

Providing assisted reproduction to physically challenged or medically ill individuals (HIV, end-stage renal/hepatic/cardiac disease, etc.) has been a concern due to the following reasons:
- In conditions where there is a risk of transmitting the disease/disability to the child.
- When there is an increased risk of adverse pregnancy outcomes that can arise due to the pregnant woman's disability.
- The concerns related to child-rearing.

Earlier, physicians have denied infertility treatment to HIV-infected individuals. But with the introduction of potent antiretroviral therapy [Highly active antiretroviral therapy (HAART)], denying treatment may be unjustified. The only counter-argument for this notion is that the physician is not only responsible for fulfilling the needs of his patient, but also responsible for the well-being of the child born through ART.

Severe Male Factor Infertility

In men with severe male factor infertility, there is a concern about transmitting underlying genetic abnormalities to the offspring. Y-chromosome microdeletions are seen in approximately 10% of men with nonobstructive azoospermia or severe oligozoospermia.[9]

Surgical sperm retrieval and intracytoplasmic sperm injection (ICSI) allow these men to father a child. The ethical issues that can arise are that their male children will also have Y-chromosome microdeletions leading to infertility issues. Another condition which has an autosomal recessive transmission is congenital bilateral absence of the vas deferens due to mutations in *CFTR* gene. There can be a transmission of this defect and also an increased risk of cystic fibrosis in the child in certain circumstances. The concern about propagating male infertility by offering sperm retrieval and ICSI in case of men who have genetically inheritable conditions is a subject of debate.

In most of these instances, an integrated approach involving a multidisciplinary medical team, hospital ethics committee, and couples with their families would be able to assess an individual's desire versus feasibility.

THE EMBRYO

An embryo is the early stage of fetal development. Following fertilization of the oocyte by a spermatozoon, and up to 8 weeks after fertilization, the conceptus is called embryo.

Embryo Handling and Rights

"What is life and when does life begin?" is a question most often asked but never answered completely. The common belief is that "Life begins at conception." If so, does the embryo have life and rights similar to those of human beings? If we agree that the embryo has life, is it ethical to destroy embryos or use them for research purposes? Some countries such as Germany do not allow freezing of embryos except in emergency situations like failed or difficult embryo transfers or at the 2PN (pronuclear) stage. Such scenarios would force couples to destroy excess embryos generated through IVF. Suggestions for such situations would entail the use of minimal ovarian stimulation in order to obtain only the desired number of embryos. However, responses to ovarian stimulation are not always predictable and can result in paucity or excess of embryos. In a country like India, where consideration has to be given to the socio-economic background of patients, this kind of approach which might necessitate multiple ART cycles may not be beneficial to patients.

Number of Embryos to be Transferred

Multiple pregnancies are a known complication of ART. Judicious use of hormonal ovarian stimulation can reduce the incidence of multiple pregnancies in ovulation induction and IUI cycles. In IVF/ICSI, the multiple pregnancy rates largely depend on the number of embryos transferred, except for the infrequent occurrence of monozygotic twinning after single embryo transfer. Although there is an improvement in pregnancy rate and outcome after selective single embryo transfer, there are IVF programs which transfer multiple embryos in order to increase pregnancy rates and sometimes as per the desire of couples. An increase in multiple pregnancy rates, with an increase in twin pregnancies from 1 to 31% and triplets from 0 to 6%, has been reported. Paradoxically, when more than three embryos were transferred, though there was no increase in the pregnancy rates, there was a significant increase in twin (45%) and triplet (16%) pregnancies.[10] Hence, the justification of transferring multiple embryos in the light of various consequences such as preterm birth, small for gestational age babies, increased risk of perinatal morbidity and mortality, maternal complications, and socioeconomic strain on the families should be considered before the transfer. Although one can resort to selective fetal reduction, this procedure carries its own hazards and should be avoided as a solution to the problem of multiple pregnancies. Studies reveal that complications such as preterm delivery correlate most often with the starting number of sacs than the finishing number,[11] which creates ethical dilemmas arising from multiple embryo transfer.

Counseling regarding the risk of multiple pregnancies following transfer of more than one embryo needs discussion with the patients: the factors that influence the success rate for that couple, success rates with the number of embryos transferred, the risk of multiple pregnancies for the same, the risks of multifetal pregnancy reduction, and the cost involved with each procedure.

Elective single-embryo transfer (e-SET) is an accepted way of mitigating multifetal gestation. However, there is discordance in the acceptance and practice of e-SET, depending on socioeconomic, ethnic, religious, and geographical conditions and available facilities. Data collected between 1978 and 2010 showed that the e-SET rates were highest in Sweden (69.4%) and least in the USA (2.8%).[12] Available data also shows a rapid increase in the number of e-SET done in the USA after 2010, though there has been a significant decline in live-birth rates when compared to two-embryo transfers.[13] In a country like India where public funding or insurance facilities are neither available nor accessible for infertility-related treatment, patients and doctors may wish to make the best of resources and transfer multiple embryos.[14]

Gender Selection

Gender selection is not permitted in India. Sex determination may be done by registered centers only to diagnose, prevent, or treat a sex-linked disorder or disease. In India, gender selection, because of female feticide and female infanticide, has led to an unbalanced sex ratio in many states as evidenced in the consecutive census until 2011. As per the census, the child sex ratio was 919 females per 1,000 males and adult sex ratio was 943 females per 1,000 males. The Pre-Natal Diagnostic Techniques (Regulation and Prevention of

Misuse) (PNDT) Act was passed by the Indian government in 1994 to stop female feticide due to the declining female sex ratio in India. Later, amendments were made to this act in 2003 and it was renamed as the Pre-Conception and Pre-Natal Diagnostic Techniques (Prohibition of Sex Selection) Act. According to this act, any form of sex selection including preimplantation genetic testing (PGT) for sex selection is illegal, except for certain prescribed indications such as sex-linked genetic diseases and other abnormalities prescribed by the Central Supervisory Board, for which procedures such as amniocentesis, chorionic villus biopsy, fetoscopy, fetal skin or organ biopsy or cordocentesis can be conducted.[15]

Preimplantation Genetic Testing for Aneuploidy (PGT-A)

Preimplantation genetic testing is permitted to screen embryos for known, heritable, or genetic diseases only in laboratories registered with individual authorities and municipal corporations as laid down by the PCPNDT body. PGT has claimed to improve pregnancy rates in ART by aiding in the selection of euploid embryos for transfer, more so in conditions such as increased maternal age and recurrent implantation failure. Even this technique is riddled with controversies. With highly sophisticated techniques, and the cost and efforts involved, the procedure does not identify an "implantable embryo." Many embryos are discarded after being tested as aneuploid embryos. It is well known that there is inherent mosaicism in human embryos and natural self-correction, and there are reports of viable healthy pregnancies even after transferring aneuploid/mosaic embryos.[16] However, this raises ethical concerns about performing a procedure that may increase the risk of cycle cancellation due to nonavailability of embryos and discarding of embryos which could have been implanted, and, the psychological effect of these on the patients.

THIRD-PARTY REPRODUCTION
Gamete Donation

In India, success with sperm donation was reported earlier than the report of the first pregnancy with oocyte donation which was reported in the mid-1980s. In spite of its established use and benefits, acceptance of gamete donation is still a decision that couples have to grapple with emotionally due to individual beliefs and family and societal pressures. This is more apparent in countries with cultural and traditional prejudices such as India.[17]

Oocyte and sperm donation guidelines vary depending on the local culture and receptiveness of the people. In Europe, Germany does not allow egg donation, while anonymous egg donation is allowed in France, Greece, Hungary, Italy, Poland, Portugal, Slovenia, and Spain and non-anonymous donation in Austria, Finland, Netherlands, Sweden, and UK. Belgium supports both anonymous and non-anonymous egg donation.[18]

Oocyte donation is indicated in conditions such as premature ovarian failure, gonadal dysgenesis including Turner syndrome, ovarian failure following chemotherapy or radiotherapy, in women who have undergone bilateral oophorectomy, and certain cases of recurrent IVF/ICSI failure where the oocyte quality was found to be compromised.[19] Oocyte donation may also be offered to women with diminished ovarian reserve or a low ovarian response, which could be a suspected or actual low response to ovarian stimulation resulting in less number and quality of oocytes or when there is a risk of transmitting a genetic condition to the offspring. Sometimes, women with endometriosis and occasionally women with polycystic ovarian syndrome (PCOS) are offered this choice even though there are studies showing comparable clinical pregnancy and live birth rates in these conditions.[20,21]

Clear guidelines have been established regarding the age of gamete donors. Considering the health consequences that can arise for the donors from oocyte donation, either during the ovarian stimulation, the IVF procedure, or after the procedure, there needs to be a finite number of times that a woman may donate eggs. But, arriving at the number of times a man may donate sperms is difficult to decide. It is difficult to keep track of the number of times gamete donation is done by an individual and it can be a challenging task. This is due to the nonavailability of a national registry and interlinking of data from centers across the country. Though it is essential that an oocyte donor should be an ever-married woman having at least one live child of her own, there are reports of unmarried girls donating oocytes for "quick money."[22] The payment may also depend on the physical appearance and educational qualifications.[23,24] If guidelines demand consent of spouse for oocyte donation, recommendations regarding the rights of unmarried girls or separated/divorced women to make a decision on donating oocytes need to be examined.

Semen donation requires relatively lesser efforts when compared to oocyte donation, and therefore there may be many volunteers for semen donation. Oocyte donation requires multiple injections, frequent visits to the ART clinic, need to undergo an invasive procedure of oocyte retrieval, and anesthesia administration and involves more complications such as hyperstimulation and procedure-related issues. Bearing these in mind, expecting altruistic oocyte donation, especially for an unknown individual, might be a "*pie in the sky*," at least for the time being in a country like India, where acceptance and awareness regarding oocyte donation are still not socially uniform. There is exploitation of donors, where women agree for oocyte donation for minimal commercial gain—*an oocyte for a dime*.[25]

Overstimulating the ovaries of donors in order to retrieve as many oocytes as possible in a single cycle is harmful to the oocyte donor. Many donors are unaware of the undesirable effects they may face after ovarian stimulation. There have also been reports of deaths due to hyperstimulation.[26,27] Monetary compensation for gamete donation, especially oocyte donation, is quite controversial. Arguments range from suggestions that gametes are the "sacred building blocks" of human life; therefore, they should not be purchased or commodified[28] to noncompensation of donors which may imply that the society does not value the significance of their contribution, despite their physical and emotional stress and the impact on their health.[29] A fixed financial remuneration may also motivate egg donation from genuine sources and reduce the exploitation and any undesired practices to a certain extent.

Surrogacy

Surrogacy is a method of ART wherein a woman carries a pregnancy for another couple. It involves complex ethical, moral, and social issues. There are two types of surrogacy—traditional or gestational surrogacy. Traditional surrogacy is where the surrogate mother undergoes artificial insemination with the intended father's sperm, where the surrogate is also the genetic mother. This method is currently not in use. Gestational surrogacy involves placing the embryo of the intending couple in the womb of a surrogate mother. In layman's parlance, it is referred to as "renting a womb."

The guidelines for surrogacy and the selection of a surrogate mother also vary in different countries and are similar to guidelines laid down for gamete donation. Earlier, commercial surrogacy was allowed in India and was available for Overseas Citizens of India (OCIs) and People of Indian Origin (PIOs). India was considered to be the "*hub*" *of surrogacy* due to good and cost-effective medical facilities, satisfactory infrastructure, and availability of potential surrogates with Indian social values.[30] A study done by the United Nations around that time estimated the surrogacy industry to be worth more than $400 million a year was being practiced by over 3,000 fertility clinics across India.[31] In order to prevent exploitation of surrogate mothers by foreign nationals, the Government of India with the assistance of the Indian Council of Medical Research (ICMR) has formulated rules and guidelines. It is an observation that women from developing countries who are serving the role of surrogates are more vulnerable to financial and other forms of exploitation.

Altruistic Surrogacy

In altruistic surrogacy, earlier only a close relative of the intending couple was permitted to be a surrogate mother. The ensuing danger could be that the surrogate mother may be made to pretend as a close relative to the intending couple, a situation that may not be proven otherwise. This may again lead to financial exploitation of the surrogate woman. The latest bill has considered this and has permitted that any willing woman may opt to be a surrogate mother.

Ethical Aspects

The guidelines or laws governing the practice of surrogacy are being revised constantly. The major task and mission are to protect the rights of the commissioning couple, the surrogate mother, and the child born through surrogacy. There are arguments that the surrogate mothers are commodified, because most often the intending couples are affluent, whereas the surrogate mothers belong to the lower socioeconomic group. The argument against this is that women have the right to choose or decide what they can do. As per the Surrogacy (Regulation) Bill 2019, only married couples who are Indian nationals are eligible for surrogacy. The length of the marriage has to be for at least 5 years. Another condition is that they should not have a child who is born biologically or is adopted or has been created through surrogacy. The surrogate mother should be related to the intending couple and should be an ever-married woman between the age of 25 and 35 years, and, have a child of her own. Subsequently in 2020, the Surrogacy (Regulation) Bill, 2020, was drafted after making few amendments and was approved by the Union Cabinet on February 26, 2020. The current bill allows an intending couple with valid medical indications to opt for surrogacy irrespective of the duration of infertility. It also allows surrogacy for single women (widow or divorcee), and any "willing woman" can be a surrogate, not necessarily a close relative.[32]

Although there are guidelines for the number of embryos that can be transferred, multiple embryos may be transferred by some clinics in order to hasten the successful outcome for the intending parents. This can result in complications for the surrogate. Clear guidelines on compensation to the surrogate in case of complications during pregnancy, delivery, and in the postpartum period, need to be defined and awareness should be created regarding the physical and emotional stress the surrogate mothers may be challenged with during pregnancy and in the postpartum period.

Child's Rights

The rights of the child born through surrogacy are almost universally accepted. The child born through the procedure of surrogacy shall be the biological child of the intending couple and will therefore be entitled to all rights and privileges under any law. The intending couple shall accept the child irrespective of the physical or mental status of the child or the sex of the child. They shall not abandon the child for any reason whatsoever, including reasons such as genetic or birth defects or any other medical condition in the child.

Rights of the Child Born through ART

The child born through ART will be considered the biological child of the couple and entitled to all rights and privileges

under the law. A donor shall not assert any parental rights on the child. The questions that arise are as follows:
- Do children have the rights to sue the parents in case of "wrongful birth" following assisted reproduction?
- Do children have a right to know their biological parent even if the foster parents decide against it?
- Do the children have a right to know their parents when the gamete donors are against revealing their identity?
- Will voluntary donation be viable if the identity of the donor is disclosed, as several surveys have revealed that the majority of gamete donors would prefer nondisclosure of their identity?[33]

UTERINE TRANSPLANTATION

The last decade has been a witness to this emerging technology. The fertility options that were available for women with absolute uterine factor infertility were adoption or surrogacy until 2014, when the first child was born following uterine transplantation in Sweden. Uterine transplantation raises issues of being temporary, non-lifesaving, experimental, and expensive. The risks involved with the surgical procedure remain for both the donor and the recipient, and immunosuppression for the recipient also poses significant challenges. The child/fetus will also be exposed to immunosuppressive drugs throughout its intrauterine life. All these aspects should be considered before opting for this procedure in the light of established alternatives available such as adoption or surrogacy.

DESIGNER BABIES

A designer baby is one whose genetic make-up has been designed by genetic engineering to ensure the presence or absence of a particular gene or characteristics. The first designer baby, Adam Nash, was born in October 2000 in the USA. The parents and sister Molly had Fanconi anemia. PGD and HLA antigen testing was done to choose the embryo which would be a suitable match as a donor for the affected sibling who required cord blood stem cell transplantation.[34] In 2002, HFEA, UK, gave permission and in 2003 the first designer baby in UK was born to provide cord blood stem cells for sibling. This concept of "savior siblings" has provided hope for children with life-threatening genetic diseases. Yet, all over the world there is an ongoing debate about the ethical considerations involved, such as savior siblings being treated as commodities and the resulting physical and psychological stress on these kids. Although genetic engineering was initially advocated for specific genetic diseases, it was further extrapolated to include sex selection for family balancing. Ethicists are, therefore, concerned that this may lead to the rampant creation of "designer babies" for physical traits such as eye color, skin color, height, and IQ and the excessive control the parents pose over the children's life even before they are born.[35] The other concern is the unknown long-term effects that may arise out of the genetic modifications.

POSTHUMOUS COLLECTION OF GAMETES

Posthumous collection of gametes may be done only if prior consent has been obtained from both the partners. This may be applicable only if prior consent was obtained in a terminally ill patient for posthumous retrieval of gametes or a routine consent before ART was used using stored embryos. If the death of the husband or male partner is sudden and unexpected, the wife/female partner may not be able to request for posthumous retrieval of gametes, which can become a matter of concern. Similar concerns may arise in the case of "brain dead" or comatose patients where consent may not be possible. As per Cornell's guidelines, in the absence of consent from the deceased, only the consent of the wife matters as the next of kin because she is the woman with whom the deceased had intended to have children.[36]

RELIGIOUS ISSUES IN ASSISTED REPRODUCTIVE TECHNOLOGY

Many ethicists, religious leaders, and theologians object to ART. They feel that doctors and scientists are either playing God, meddling with nature, playing with life, or creating life. There are many physicians who consider that most treatments and procedures in medicine are against nature, right from wearing spectacles to organ transplantation. Yet, we continue to do it either to save lives or to improve the quality of life. This may be applicable to ARTs too. This issue is evolving from time to time and needs constant debate to reach a consensus.

ETHICAL ISSUES IN ASSISTED REPRODUCTIVE TECHNOLOGY

Though most of the issues related to specific conditions like embryo handling and research, maintaining confidentiality, and compensation have been mentioned in the respective sections, there are many more issues that practitioners of ART are faced with in day-to-day practice. Comprehensive counseling should include medical, procedural, societal, and economic aspects of ART. The possibility of failure of treatment needs to be explained to the couple. The physician may only act as a guide for the patients and not as the decision-maker. The couple should be given adequate time to read the informed consent form and then encouraged to make their own decisions. The consent form should include details about the procedures, the number of embryos to be transferred, willingness for anesthesia and complications, and storage of gametes or embryos. Profit-driven unethical medical practice has been a concern for quite some time.[37] The virtues and moral values of the physician play a major role in ethical practice. In an emerging field like ART, these values along with strict regulations from the authorities will help in preventing abuse or exploitation of the most vulnerable and desperate group of patients, the involved third party, and harm to the progeny.

ICMR GUIDELINES AND THE ART REGULATIONS BILL

The ICMR issued guidelines in 2005 and then in 2014 and 2017, for the accreditation, supervision, and regulation of ART clinics. Currently, these guidelines are not legally binding.[38,39] The Union Cabinet in India approved the ART Regulations Bill 2020, the Surrogacy Regulation Bill 2020, and the Medical Termination of Pregnancy Amendment Bill 2020. These services require regulations to protect women and children from exploitation. The regulations are constantly revised to accommodate the changes in the expectations of the society and the evolving technological advances in this field, keeping in mind the welfare of all parties involved and that of the child born through these techniques.[40]

CONCLUSION

Assisted reproduction is an ethical minefield. The desire and desperation of the couple for a baby can be subject to exploitation. This field of medicine has its share of unethical practices. In addition to the existing procedures to achieve parenthood, the evolving technological advances such as gene editing and mitochondrial transfer will generate further dilemmas and ethical issues. The physician plays a pivotal role in ethical practice. Strict regulations and implementation of the same from apex bodies such as ICMR would mitigate exploitation of the infertile couple who tend to be weak and vulnerable members of the society. As always, "Primum non nocere" should be the motto of the ART specialists, bearing in mind the best interest of the couple, children, and the third party involved.

Authors declare no conflicts of interest.

REFERENCES

1. Pandiyan N. Embryo sex selection: a social comment on the article by Malpani and Malpani. Reprod Biomed Online. 2001;4(1):9-10.
2. ESHRE (European Society for Human Reproduction and Embryology) (2018). ART Fact Sheet. ESHRE Press Information. [online] Available from: https://www.eshre.eu/Press-Room/Resources [Last accessed October, 2021].
3. Programme of Action of the International Conference on Population and Development, Cairo, 1994. New York: United Nations; 1995: paragraph 7.2-7.3.
4. Pandiyan N, Puvithra T. Is reproduction a fundamental right? A clinical, ethical and personal perspective. Chettinad Health City Med J. 2017;6(4):152-3.
5. Pennings G. Ethical issues of infertility treatment in developing countries. ESHRE Monogr. 2008;2008(1):15-20.
6. Zegers-Hochschild F, Adamson GD, Dyer S, Racowsky C, de Mouzon J, Sokol R, et al. The International Glossary on Infertility and Fertility Care, 2017. Fertil Steril. 2017;108(3):393-406.
7. NICE. (2004). Fertility: assessment and treatment for people with fertility problems. National Collaborating Centre for Women's and Children's Health for the National Institute of Clinical Excellence. London: RCOG Press; 2004.
8. Krajewska A. Access of single women to fertility treatment: A case of incidental discrimination? Med Law Rev. 2015; 23(4):620-45.
9. Waseem AS, Singh V, Makker GC, Trivedi S, Mishra G, Singh K, et al. AZF deletions in Indian populations: original study and meta-analyses. J Assist Reprod Genet. 2020;37(2):459-69.
10. The ESHRE Task Force on Ethics and Law; 6. Ethical issues related to multiple pregnancies in medically assisted procreation. Hum Reprod. 2003;18(9):1976-9.
11. Evans MI, Krivchenia EL, Gelber SE, Wapner RJ. Selective reduction. Clin Perinatol. 2003;30(1):103-11.
12. Maheshwari A, Griffiths S, Bhattacharya S. Global variations in the uptake of single embryo transfer. Hum Reprod Update. 2011;17(1):107-20.
13. Gleicher N, Mochizuki L, Barad DH. Time associations between U.S. birth rates and add-ons to IVF practice between 2005-2016. Reprod Biol Endocrinol. 2021;19(1):110.
14. Hema V, Gopinath PM, Gayathri Devi SS. Knowledge, attitudes and concerns towards elective single embryo transfer (eSET) in couples undergoing fresh/frozen embryo transfer cycles in Asian population. Fertil Steril. 2019;112(Suppl 3):E379-80.
15. Bhaktwani A. The PC-PNDT act in a nutshell. Indian J Radiol Imaging. 2012;22(2):133-4.
16. Fragouli E, Alfarawati S, Spath K, Babariya D, Tarozzi N, Borini A, et al. Analysis of implantation and ongoing pregnancy rates following the transfer of mosaic diploid-aneuploid blastocysts. Hum Genet. 2017;136(7):805-19.
17. Banerjee K, Singla B. Acceptance of donor eggs, donor sperms, or donor embryos in Indian infertile couples. J Hum Reprod Sci. 2018;11(2):169-71.
18. ESHRE Fact Sheets 3 (2017). Egg donation. [online] Available from: https://www.eshre.eu/-/media/sitecore-files/Press-room/Resources/3-Egg- donation.pdf [Last accessed October 2021].
19. National Collaborating Centre for Women's and Children's Health (UK). Fertility: Assessment and Treatment for People with Fertility Problems. London: Royal College of Obstetricians & Gynaecologists; 2013 Feb. (NICE Clinical Guidelines, No. 156.) 18, Oocyte donation.
20. Bishop LA, Gunn J, Jahandideh S, Devine K, Decherney AH, Hill MJ. Endometriosis does not impact live-birth rates in frozen embryo transfers of euploid blastocysts. Fertil Steril. 2021;115(2):416-22.
21. Tang K, Wu L, Luo Y, Gong B. In vitro fertilization outcomes in women with polycystic ovary syndrome: a meta-analysis. Eur J Obstet Gynecol Reprod Biol. 2021;259:146-52.
22. Bawa R (2010). Delhi girls donating eggs for quick money. India Today. [online] Available from: https://www.indiatoday.in/india/north/story/delhi-girls-donating-eggs-for-quick-money-80214-2010-08-11 [Last accessed October, 2021].
23. Beeson D (2018). Egg selling in India. Centre for Genetics and Society. Biopolitical Times. [online] Available from: https://www.geneticsandsociety.org/biopolitical-times/egg-selling-india [Last accessed October, 2021].
24. Rao CS (2017). The more beautiful the female egg donor, the higher the price they can command. The Times of India. [online] Available from: https://timesofindia.indiatimes.com/city/hyderabad/the-more-beautiful-the-female-egg-donor-the-higher-the-price-they-can-command/articleshow/58587401.cms.

25. Vora P (2018). 'No other way to earn money': Why women from poor families become egg donors for infertile couples. Scroll.in. [online]. Available from: https://scroll.in/pulse/881658/no-other-way-to-earn-money-why-women-from-poor-families-become-egg-donors-for-infertile-couples [Last accessed October, 2021].
26. The Indian Express (2014). Egg donor's death: Internal bleeding, ovaries severely enlarged, says report. [online] Available from: https://indianexpress.com/article/india/india-others/egg-donors-death-internal-bleeding-ovaries-severely-enlarged-says-report/.
27. Dhayalkar S (2018). The curious case of 17-year-old egg donor from Saki Naka who died over 7 years ago. The Indian Express. [online] Available from: https://indianexpress.com/article/cities/mumbai/the-curious-case-of-17-year-old-egg-donor-from-saki-naka-who-died-over-7-years-ago-5070576/.
28. Cohen CB. Selling bits and pieces of humans to make babies: The gift of the magi revisited. J Med Philos. 1999;24(3):288-306.
29. Ethics Committee of the American Society for Reproductive Medicine. Financial compensation of oocyte donors. Fertil Steril. 2007;88(2):305-9.
30. Patel NH, Jadeja YD, Bhadarka HK, Patel MN, Patel NH, Sodagar NR. Insight into different aspects of surrogacy practices. J Hum Reprod Sci. 2018;11(3):212-8.
31. Bhalla N, Thapliyal M (2013). India seeks to regulate its booming surrogacy industry. Medscape Reuters Health News. 2013. [online] Available from: https://www.reuters.com/article/us-india-surrogates/india-seeks-to-regulate-its-booming-rent-a-womb-industry-idUSBRE98T07F20130930 [Last accessed October, 2021].
32. Bhumitra D, Yash T (2020). Analysis of the Surrogacy (Regulation) Bill, 2020. Indian Law J. [online] Available from: https://www.indialawjournal.org/analysis-of-the-surrogacy-regulation-bill.php [Last accessed October, 2021].
33. Khamsi F, Endman MW, Lacanna IC, Wong J. Some psychological aspects of oocyte donation from known donors on altruistic basis. Fertil Steril.1997;68:323-7.
34. Verlinsky Y, Rechitsky S, Schoolcraft W, Strom C, Kuliev A. Preimplantation diagnosis for Fanconi anemia combined with HLA matching. JAMA. 2001;285(24):3130-3.
35. Sheldon S, Wilkinson S. Should selecting saviour siblings be banned? J Med Ethics. 2004;30:533-7.
36. Sikary AK, Murty OP, Bardale RV. Postmortem sperm retrieval in context of developing countries of Indian subcontinent. J Hum Reprod Sci. 2016;9(2):82-5.
37. Macklin R. Reproductive technologies in developing countries. Bioethics.1995;9:276-82.
38. Indian Council of Medical Research (2010). Ministry of Health and Family Welfare. The Assisted Reproductive Technologies (Regulation) Bill – 2010 (Draft). [online] Available from: https://main.icmr.nic.in/sites/default/files/guidelines/ART%20REGULATION%20Draft%20Bill1.pdf.
39. PRS Legislative Research. The Surrogacy (Regulation) Bill, 2019. [online] Available from: http://prsindia.org/billtrack/surrogacy-regulation-bill-2019 [Last accessed October, 2021].
40. Press Information Bureau, Government of India. Cabinet approves the Assisted Reproductive Technology Regulation Bill 2020. Path breaking measures taken to protect women's reproductive rights. [Press release] ART Regulation Bill 2020. Press Information Bureau. Delhi, 2020. [online] Available from: https://pib.gov.in/PressReleseDetail.aspx?PRID=1603649 [Last accessed October, 2021].

CHAPTER 8

Status of Traditional Medicine: Integrative and Ethical Perspectives in India

Nandini K Kumar, Pradeep Dua

ABSTRACT

The traditional Indian medicine (TIM) is based on the epistemology of the interactions and relationship of cosmos on human body, mind, and spirit. Millennia-old clinical experience, guided by theoretical substratum and texts, was transmitted across generations, until college education in TIM emerged. In contrast to the biomedicine (BM), which is based on universally applicable and scientifically validated principles of diagnosis and treatment, TIM characterizes individual patient-centric diagnosis and specific treatment modalities. As a consequence, the so-called "gold standard"—randomized controlled clinical trials (RCTs) for scientifically validating the safety and efficacy of these time-tested TIM are quite often not suitable for their real-life evaluation due to the biological complexities of the individual host-disease interacting responses. To adopt a bedside to bench research and validation of the ancient science of TIM, the dedicated approaches to pharmacoepidemiology, robust observational studies and reverse pharmacology have been proposed and used in India. The evolution of guidelines and regulations to govern research on TIM—classical as well as proprietary Ayurvedic, Siddha, and Unani drugs, and other herbal/herbo-mineral formulations—have guided research in TIM by addressing the challenges related to standardization of the raw drug and the finished product, nondrug therapy as well as clinical research protocols, and associated ethical considerations.

In order to promote global acceptance of these codified systems of TIM, the Ministry of AYUSH, Government of India, is endeavoring to meet these challenges through strengthening the standards of pharmacopoeia and drug development and has concerted these efforts at the national and international level through the Bureau of Indian Standards (BIS) and International Organization for Standardization (ISO).

INTRODUCTION

"Life is the combination of body, senses, mind, and reincarnating soul. Ayurveda is the sacred science of life, beneficial to humans both in this world and the world beyond."

—Caraka

"A physician without a knowledge of Astrology has no right to call himself a physician."

—Hippocrates

The above-mentioned quotes suggest that the ancient founders of medicine did believe in the cosmophysiological effect of natural forces on human body, mind, and spirit. Mystical and spiritual insights were gained about interrelationship between the macrocosm and microcosm up to atomic and quantum levels involved in the body.[1,2] The TIM got refined over centuries through intelligent observations of animal and human behavior, when healthy or ill. Ancient scriptures of Indian philosophy in the presystemic era were the *Vedas, Upanishads, and epics*. Out of the four *Vedas*, two refer to Ayurveda, namely, *Rig Veda* and *Atharva Veda*. While *Rig Veda* provides few references related to medicine, a major part of *Atharva Veda*, of which Ayurveda is a branch (*Upaveda*) describes treatment modalities for diseases affecting body[3,4]. Ayurveda and Siddha medicines are stated to have divine origins, from Brahma and Shiva respectively. Five elements of nature were recognized to have influence on health as sensors and effectors combined with mind; these are *Aakasha* (entity responsible for space), *Vaayu* (entity responsible for movement), *Agni* (entity responsible for heat), *Jala* (entity responsible for fluidity), and *Prithvi* (entity responsible for hardness), the *Pancha Mahabhutas*. Since Unani medicine originated from Greece, it imbibed Hellenistic philosophy of belief in four elements of nature—(1) air, (2) fire, (3) water, and (4) earth—affecting health. Sowa-Rigpa (Tibetan/Amchi medicine) which has recently been recognized by the Indian Government, practices a combination of local *Amchi* treatment and Ayurveda.

The fundamental difference of these TIM systems from BM is that the latter, which is only >200 years old, emphasizes on only the physical dimension of health and hence has not given the expected relief from behavioral, emotional, or spiritual factors causing disease.[5] These are the very factors which have important roles in TIM. Therefore, the ethical issues and challenges faced by TIM in research are quite different and difficult in creating scientific evidence of their efficacy. Before describing further about the research in TIM, for a better understanding of the theme of this chapter, we may consider the classification by the World Health Organization (WHO) into three categories given below as traditional, complementary, and herbal medicine.[6]

- **Traditional medicine**: Traditional medicine (TM) is the sum total of the knowledge, skills, and practices based on the theories, beliefs, and experiences indigenous to different cultures, whether these are explicable or not, used in the maintenance of health as well as in the prevention, diagnosis, improvement, or treatment of physical and mental illness.
- **Complementary medicine**: The terms "complementary medicine" or "alternative medicine" refer to a broad set of healthcare practices that are not part of that country's own tradition or conventional medicine and are not fully integrated into the dominant healthcare system. They are often used interchangeably with traditional medicine in some countries.
- **Herbal medicines**: Herbal medicines include herbs, herbal materials, herbal preparations, and finished herbal products that contain active ingredients, parts of plants, or other plant materials, or combinations.

The term "traditional medicine" is usually used when referring to Africa, Latin America, Asia, and/or the Western Pacific, whereas the same is termed as "complementary and alternative medicine" (CAM/CM) in Europe, North America, Canada, and Australia. WHO has also supported activities to streamline concepts related to R&D and practice of traditional medicine. Alternative terms used for BM include modern medicine, conventional medicine, orthodox medicine, allopathy, or Western medicine. In this chapter, to differentiate the traditional Indian medicine from all the other terms mentioned above, the term "TIM" will be used henceforth in place of TM.

In India, Ayurveda, Siddha, Unani (ASU), and nondrug interventions such as Yoga and Naturopathy are the recognized systems of TIM. These systems along with Homoeopathy are controlled by the Ministry of AYUSH. To this list Sowa-Rigpa got added in 2012. All these traditional medicine systems, which are codified, are based on the concept of individualized treatment. Folklore or ethnic practices of local communities or tribals are noncodified and therefore, go quite often unnoticed for their value. However, National Innovation Foundation (NIF), Ahmedabad, now a part of Department of Science and Technology (DST), has done pioneering work in compiling innovative traditional knowledge of herbals used by individuals or communities at grassroots level and validating some of the promising claims. The prior informed consent is obtained by NIF to protect this noncodified knowledge for compensation in case the research leads to new discovery. The Foundation for Revitalization in Local Health Tradition (FRLHT), Bengaluru has also carried out a lot of research on similar aspects through University of Transdisciplinary Health Sciences and Technology (TDU). However, the efforts are generally lacking for getting such claims scientifically validated for creating evidence of their safety and efficacy.

In the codified systems, the traditional medical practitioners follow their classical texts, which reflect not only the wisdom of the ancient gurus (teachers) but also their meticulous observations. Their time-tested recorded clinical observations and experiences were debated between teacher and students or fellow physicians for further refinement of practice guidelines. Even today there are efforts to re-establish the facts using modern scientific tools. The ancient practitioners had apparently taken note of characteristics of a person's constitution (*Prakriti*), causes (*Nidana*), pathogenesis (*samprapti*), state of *doshas* (predominance of Vata, Pitta, and Kapha), stage of the disease (*Shatkriyakala*), suitable and unsuitable diet and lifestyles (*Pathya-apathya*) etc., while documenting the classical compendia. This innate strength of Ayurveda through reverse pharmacology,[7,8] Prakriti-genomics/ (Ayurgenomics) and pharmacogenomics may help us understand the molecular basis of individual variations in therapeutic responses.[9,10] For several health challenges, this may increase TIMs scope of predictive and personalized medicine. Systems biology is another concept of modern science, which is being applied to Ayurveda, to study body responses.[2,8] Systems Ayurveda has also been proposed to have an integral perspective on the vast subject.[11] The improved biotechnology tools for assessing the objective markers of safety and efficacy can generate more acceptable evidence through clinical and basic research in TIM. This has created a worldwide interest in rekindling drug discovery from clinical experience in TIM.[12]

The global interest in alternative treatment has motivated the dynamic TIM practitioners to document and scientifically validate treatment regimens for global acceptance. This is not only for scholarly understanding and enriching translation in application but may also augment global trade. In 2002, WHO launched a strategy to assist countries for promotion of safe, effective, and affordable traditional medicine.[13] The strategies included: (i) developing national policies for the evaluation and regulation of TM/CAM practices; (ii) creating a stronger evidence based on the safety, efficacy, and quality of the TM/CAM products and practices; (iii) ensuring that TM/CAM including essential herbal medicines are available and affordable; (iv) promoting use of TM/CAM by providers and consumers in a scientifically sound manner; and (v) documenting traditional medicines and herbal remedies. Later, repeated surveys were conducted by WHO which showed that 88% of member states (170 in number) have developed policies, laws, regulations, education, programs, and offices for traditional medicine and complementary medicine on a formal scale.[14] The survey also records that 34 member states include traditional or herbal medicines in their list of essential medicines and >90 member states use Ayurveda, while 110 use herbals.

STATUS OF TRADITIONAL INDIAN MEDICINE IN INDIA

As in most developing countries, 80% of the Indian population resides in rural areas. Villages in India still lack proper and affordable health care, so the rural population prefer TIM because of several reasons inter alia their faith in TIM, self-medication of home remedies, and out of necessity and easy access. There is also a growing trend to use natural products and TIM amongst the urban population, due to a global shift toward preventive medicine and holistic health.

On 9th November 2014, a separate Ministry of AYUSH (Ayurveda, Yoga, Naturopathy, Unani, Siddha, Sowa-Rigpa, and Homoeopathy) was set-up to promote TIM. As a part of several innovative initiatives of the Government of India, a centralized web-based portal, National AYUSH Morbidity and Standardized Terminologies Electronic Portal (NAMASTE Portal), was launched in 2017 for collection of Standardized Ayurveda, Siddha, and Unani Terminologies and morbidity statistics from AYUSH institutions in the country. The AYUSH Morbidity Codes in the portal have been interlinked to WHO-ICD 10/11. In 2018, a comprehensive electronic health record system, namely, AYUSH Hospital Management Information System (A-HMIS), was launched to enable patients to seek standardized care from AYUSH facilities which is documented digitally on a real time basis. The revised National Health Policy on Indian Systems of Medicine and Homoeopathy (ISM&H), 2017[15] endorsed the 2002 Policy about bringing the traditional systems of medicine to the mainstream of health care through developing strategies for capacity building in human resources and infrastructure, and promoting medical pluralism. Improvement of cultivation, development, and quality control of herbal drugs is under the purview of the National AYUSH Mission (NAM) and National Medicinal Plant Board. In December, 2017, the Ministry of AYUSH has also implemented the Central Sector Scheme of Pharmacovigilance of ASU&H Drugs through a three-tier network for documentation and reporting of misleading advertisements pertaining to AYUSH systems as well as adverse events (AEs) pertaining to TIM, their documentation, and analysis thereby facilitating further regulatory action, if necessary. The Scheme is functional since June, 2018. Pharmacopoeial standards and monographs for drugs in AYUSH systems have enabled Good manufacturing practices (GMPs) compliant manufacture of products of these systems for better quality maintenance.

Other progressive collaborative initiatives of the Ministry of AYUSH include accreditation of some AYUSH Hospitals/Panchakarma clinics and daycare treatment centers by the National Accreditation Board for Hospitals and Healthcare Providers (NABH) facilitating, administration of standardized care, and admissibility for insurance coverage and reimbursement. Another important activity is that of the BIS pertaining to formulation of Indian Standards for terminology of Ayurveda and Yoga, Yoga accessories, panchakarma equipment and ingredients of ASU formulations. Several other projects of BIS including development of national standards for herbal extracts and panchagavya ingredients including cow ghee are in the pipeline. Two proposals from India including "Health Informatics—introduction to Ayurveda" and "Health Informatics—categorial structures for preparation of Ayurvedic medicinal water in Ayurveda" have been accepted in the program of work of ISO TC 215 (WG 10) for formulation of International deliverables in the ISO. Other initiatives are data mining, analytics, and artificial intelligence for traditional knowledge inspired drug discovery and food as medicine.

In April 2020, the Ministry of AYUSH constituted seven "Interdisciplinary AYUSH Research and Development Task Force" working groups to initiate, coordinate, and monitor R&D activities related to COVID-19 disease in the AYUSH sector with interagency collaboration as a solidarity effort. Presently, NITI (National Institution for Transforming India) Aayog has constituted a Committee to formulate an Integrative Health Policy with four working groups for core areas of Education, Research, Clinical Practice, and Public Health and Administration. Under this, it is planned to create an integrated curriculum of modern medicine, Ayurveda, and Yoga in some chosen medical undergraduate colleges which will hopefully be implemented by 2030. This is a challenging step to promote "One Nation–One Healthcare" concept by the Government. This can provide the needed synergy in pluralistic health care also in demand in the developed world like Europe,[16,17] Australia, and other Western countries like US and Canada where already there is a greater acceptance of the patient-centric traditional medicine care.

In India, the term alternative systems of medicine (ASM) connotes a different meaning and is recognized by the Government only if it satisfies the essential and desirable criteria as laid down by the Standing Committee of Experts to examine claims of ASM set-up by the Ministry of Health and Family Welfare. Out of 16 such claims made at that time only hypnotherapy and acupuncture have been recognized as therapies requiring professionally trained practitioners to practice them as per Government Order in 2003.

FUNDING FOR RESEARCH ON TRADITIONAL MEDICINE

In spite of concerns regarding the lack of regulation of complementary practice, the House of Lords, UK recognized the increasing use of traditional medicine in its report on alternative and complementary medicine. The Prince of Wales had even called for a £10 million investment in such research in 2000.[18] Funding for development of traditional medicine has been growing in the US under the aegis of the National Center for Complementary and Integrative Health (NCCIH). For 2021, the budget estimate sanctioned by Congress is for $124.5 million.[19] Between the year 1999 and 2018, the growth of traditional medicine research institutes of member states of WHO has been from 19 to 75.[14]

The Indian Government allocated ₹ 2970.30 crores to the Ministry of AYUSH for the year 2021–22 marking a 40% hike to current year's budget of ₹ 2122.08 crores. There were 822 ongoing research projects as on March 2020.[20] Besides the Ministry, various Government research institutions such as Indian Council of Medical Research (ICMR), DST, and Department of Biotechnology (DBT), and private sectors including philanthropic foundations have been undertaking R&D on herbals and herbo-minerals, but there is no nationwide centralized data to show a consolidated figure for the funds spent by the above-mentioned domains to provide a perspective on the proportions of the public and private funds spent on the TIM research.

MEDICAL ETHICS IN INDIAN SYSTEMS OF MEDICINE

The tradition of Siddha and Ayurveda existed from Vedic times, but from 3000 BC to 2nd century AD onward. We have evidence of manuscripts and texts—prominent ones of Siddha being *Thylavarga Churukkam* and *Agathiyar Sillaraikkovai*, and those of Ayurveda, classics such as *Caraka Samhita, Sushruta Samhita, Ashtanga Sangraha*, etc. These texts state that physicians should follow code of conduct and be compassionate and honest. There was a maxim that the ideal therapy for a disease should not be one, which would lead to expression of another disease—iatrogenic disorders. In Siddha, additional emphasis is laid on good health for fulfilling one's Dharma (spiritual attainment). *Agathiyar Sillaraikkovai* of Siddha medicine states that the physician should protect the patient just as how the eyelid would protect one's eye. In Ayurveda, judicious usage of *Daivavyapashraya* (the mystic and spiritual healing), *Yuktivyapashraya* (logic) and *Sattvavajaya* (psychotherapy) chikitsa coupled with *Achar Rasayana* (ethical and healthy lifestyle) is advised.

The compassionate attitude of the physicians was reflected when deciding a treatment in the best interest of the patient, but due to the paternalistic societal norms of those times, the patient's consent was considered immaterial.[21] Both Siddha and Unani systems also did not consider patient preferences. *Kamilussanah,* a 10th century AD book of Unani medicine, also reflects the same paternalism in the code of conduct for physicians.[22] However, according to *Sushruta Samhita,* if surgical intervention of uncertain outcome was required to prevent death, permission to do so was to be sought from the king.[23] Same approach is described in *Caraka Samhita* too stating that in emergency condition, if there was doubt that the treatment had the possibility of causing more harm, permission from the relatives/community (well-wishers) should be sought.[24] *Arthasastra* of 3rd Century BC mentions that capital punishment would be given to the physician, who without prior permission has done major surgery which has resulted in death.[25] Existence of quack *vaidyas* were also described then and the state was expected to condemn and ban such imposters. Egyptian papyri of 16th century BC also state that if the patient died due to the physician transgressing the rules, then the physician had to pay with his own life. The Ayurvedic texts also cautioned that physicians should refrain from getting into controversy with the institution/state.

ETHICAL GUIDELINES AND REGULATIONS

Ethical considerations in Ayurveda were ingrained in all the texts which were followed religiously in the long tradition of clinical practice.[25] According to WHO, registration of traditional medicine practitioners and number of member states with traditional medicine policy and regulations have increased from earlier years.[14] Since 2011, in European Union which is divided regarding import of traditional medicine by regulatory authorities, countries such as UK and Germany allow import of traditional medicines only as dietary supplements to be consumed as a tonic, whereas, Italy, France, and Belgium import it for treatment of disease. The European Union (EU), through the Traditional Herbal Medicinal Products Directive (THMPD), Food Supplements Directive (FSD), and the Pharmaceutical Legislative Review (medicines for human use directive), permits import of only those formulations which are safe and meet quality control standards, have been in use for 30 years outside EU, and in the European market for 15 years. This was mainly due to the scare created by some, that such formulations have not undergone rigorous clinical trials as required by the respective foreign regulating agencies. Moreover, the situation jumped from the frying pan into the fire over the publication in *JAMA* of the alleged toxic content of metallic ingredients of some Ayurvedic preparations.[26] Globally, most of the pharmacopoeial standards pertain to single plant extracts or extracts of very few herbs in compound formulations where the contents are in fixed combinations. These developments have restricted the use of TIM, which could actually bring more benefits than projected. With respect to safety, the plant-based remedies are required to undergo the same assessment criteria that are now being used for modern pharmaceutical, nutraceutical, and cosmeceutical products. Standardization and quality control for herbal or herbo-mineral preparations is required to compete in the international markets.

In India, due to the growing global interest, a number of institutions pertaining to TIM have sprung up in the private sector for health care, research, and development making it necessary that some uniform guidelines and checks are in place to prevent commercial exploitation by tall unsubstantiated claims. There are 8,954 (April, 2021) licensed ASU&H drug manufacturers in the country which are GMP compliant and monitored on regular basis.[20] Presently approximately 30 manufacturing units comply to WHO GMP norms.

All proposals for clinical research including TIM can register in the Clinical Trial Registry of India (CTRI). Since TIM research also comes under biomedical and health research, the ethics committees (ECs) reviewing TIM proposals have to register under the Department of Health Research as per regulation effective from September, 2019. Ethics committees reviewing both TIM and BM proposals have members or experts from both disciplines giving their inputs. The first independent EC in India to adopt this methodology is the Inter System Biomedica Ethics Committee (ISBEC), with multisystem experts from Bio/Modern medicine, Ayurveda, Homoeopathy, and Unani medicine functioning at Kasturba Health Society, Mumbai.[27]

Research Ethics Guidelines

The first Ethical Guidelines of ICMR, titled "Policy Statement on Ethical Considerations Involved in Research on Human Subjects" in 1980,[28] had included a paragraph on traditional medicine showing how important this area was considered even at that time. In 1996, ICMR undertook the task of revising the ethical guidelines under the Chairmanship of Hon'ble Justice MN Venkatchaliah, the Chairman of the National Human Rights Commission. Besides circulating the Draft guidelines for comments, ICMR held public debates in four metro cities between 1998 and 1999. At the public meeting held in Mumbai, it was suggested that for trials on herbal preparations, EC approval and Good clinical practice (GCP) were just as much needed as for the allopathic drugs.[29] In 2000, "Ethical Guidelines for Biomedical research on Human Subjects", included a section on research on herbal remedies after consulting the Research Councils under the erstwhile Department of ISM&H.[30] These were expanded in 2006 in the "Ethical Guidelines for Biomedical research on Human Participants",[31] incorporating again the suggestions of these Research Councils as well as the WHO recommendations. However, in the third revised National Ethical Guidelines of ICMR in 2017,[32] this section was reduced because the main responsibility of research governance in this area now rested with the Ministry of AYUSH, established in 2014. All researchers, irrespective of the medical system they belong to, have to undergo GCP and research methodology training before initiating any research. In 2013, ASU GCP Guidelines was issued on the same lines as the Indian GCP for voluntary use and in 2018, three documents, namely, General Guidelines for Drug Development of Ayurvedic formulations, Safety/Toxicity Evaluation of Ayurvedic Formulations, and Clinical Evaluation of Ayurvedic Formulations, were released for ASU researchers to keep pace with current developments in the area.[33-35]

Regulations

A Committee chaired by Col. RN Chopra made recommendations for the production and sale of Drugs and pharmaceuticals which resulted in the "Drugs Act" which was enacted in 1940 followed by Rules in 1945. To this was added Cosmetics in 1962, after which the Act was called the Drugs and Cosmetics Act (DCA). Then, ASU systems got added in 1964 and ASU drugs, patent and proprietary (P&P) drugs in 1982 (Section 3a and 3h(i) of Chapter IVA)[36] as amendments. Another category, "Phytopharmaceuticals", was notified in 2015 and is included as Rule 2 (b) in the New Drug Clinical Trial (NDCT) Rules dated March 19, 2019.

In the First schedule of DCA, the authoritative ASU texts were included to identify the classical formulations. The DCA also included testing and analysis of ASU&H drugs by trained inspectors/Government Analysts in Government specified laboratories. Later amendments included manufacturing requirements under Schedule M for Homoeopathy; Schedule T for ASU drugs; Schedule T (A) for ASU drugs containing herbo-mineral ingredients; and a qualified traditional medicine practitioner to guide production and supervise every unit manufacturing ASU drugs. A separate ASU Drug Technical Advisory Board (ASUDTAB) was constituted to advise the Indian Government on all aspects related to standardization and quality control of ASU drugs.

A separate ASU Drugs Consultative Committee (ASUDCC) comprising State Drugs Licensing Authorities was set-up under DCA for uniform administration of the Act throughout India. Manufacture and sale of certain drugs was prohibited and power was given to the Central Government to oversee this in public interest. Several good ASU&H pharmacies and drugs testing laboratories have been established since 2014 under National AYUSH Mission (NAM). The full potential of these recent Government initiatives will need some more time to feel the impact.

Several other legislations touch upon one or the other dimension of the DCA with reference to ASU&H drugs. The functional foods/nutraceuticals/health supplements fall under the purview of Food Safety and Standards Authority of India (FSSAI Act of 2020). The other Acts related to TIM/herbal formulations are the Indian Forest Act, 1927; the Drugs and

Magic Remedies (Objectionable Advertisements) Act, 1954; the Wild Life Protection Act, 1972; the Standards of Weights and Measures Act, 1976; the Narcotics and Psychotropic Substances Act, 1985; and the Biodiversity Act, 2002. The terms such as herbals (medicinal) and botanicals are not used in India. Another important step taken by the Ministry of AYUSH is to have an ASU&H Drug-related vertical in the Central Drugs Standard Control Organization (CDSCO) which is functional under the administrative control of the Drug Controller General of India (DCGI), presently termed as the Central Licensing Authority (CLA).

RESEARCH IN INDIA

The Indian Research Funding Agency (IRFA) (later known as ICMR) had been involved in traditional medicine research from its very inception in 1911 as evidenced by the significant support it gave to the pioneering work of the late Sir Ram Nath Chopra, the Father of Indian Pharmacology, in the early part of his career.[37] A unique multidisciplinary approach was adopted by ICMR in the Composite Drug Research Scheme from 1964–1970 in collaboration with the erstwhile Central Council for Ayurvedic Research and Council of Scientific and Industrial Research (CSIR) in nine "circuits" across the country, each with four units comprising Clinical Unit of Ayurvedic and Modern Medicine physicians, Pharmacognosy Unit for Botany, Chemistry Unit, and Pharmacology Unit.[38] The Medicinal Plant Unit (MPU) under GV Satyavati was compiling information on Indian Medicinal Plants which is still being continued. From 1985 onward under her guidance, ICMR was involved in conducting several multicentric disease-oriented clinical trials involving herbals in BM institutions using reverse pharmacology and an integrated approach.[39] The latter approach was initiated in late seventies by Ashok Vaidya, Antarkar et al. at CIBA Research Centre and Podar Ayurvedic Hospital, Mumbai.[7,40] Several Centers of Advanced Research were set-up by ICMR for pharmacological and clinical pharmacology research on selected traditional remedies, preclinical studies, quality control, and standardization, reverse pharmacology, and Yoga in various renowned institutions/organizations across the country. These efforts resulted in interesting hits and leads in anal fistula, diabetes, hepatitis, filariasis, urolithiasis, malaria, arthritis, and cancer. The new ICMR's program of Advanced Product Development Centers took up some of these leads for developing novel phytopharmaceuticals. ICMR's Regional Medical Research Centre at Belgaum, Karnataka was dedicated for carrying out research in traditional medicine (now known as National Institute of Traditional Medicine). In a Declaration at Chitrakoot, under the guidance of Sri Nanaji Deshmukh, the Golden Triangle Partnership (GTP) program for research was proposed by Mashelkar, Vaidya, and Mehrotra. GTP involved a collaboration of institutions of modern medicine, Ayurveda, and basic sciences.[41] Though the Department of AYUSH, CSIR, and ICMR collaborated to implement GTP for prioritized clinical areas, unfortunately this ambitious project did not reach the clinical trial stage due to technical and administrative reasons.

The other major initiative in the Government sector was under CSIR's New Millennium Indian Technology Leadership Initiative (NMITLI) to develop plant-based drugs for osteoarthritis, diabetes, and hepatitis, applying the Reverse Pharmacology path involving inter-institutional collaboration.[42] This inter-institutional program had involved the government laboratories, industrial R&D, universities, medical colleges, and research centers. CSIR, DST, and DBT have also funded projects in TIM area. Besides funding Ayurveda Biology, DST recently funded the SATYAM (Science and Technology of Yoga and Meditation) project under the Cognitive Science Research Initiative (CSRI). The AYUSH Research Councils now have many collaborative programs with biomedical or scientific institutions using integrated approach to evolve patient-centric TIM treatment. MS Baghel had initiated enlisting all the MD and PhD theses in Ayurveda which is being periodically updated.[43] There has been substantial research on the pharmacology/pharmacognosy of the medicinal plants used in TIM in academia, research institutes, and pharma research centers. There are also attempts to consolidate database on the outcomes of such R&D initiatives.

INTEGRATIVE INITIATIVES

Historically, during the early 19th century, a British physician Pardie Leucas, Director of Medical Services, initiated the idea of integration of Ayurveda and BM. In early 20th century, some eminent TIM physicians such as Mayaram Sundarji, Gananath Sen, and others advocated progressive adoption of integrative Ayurveda. In 1921, through Tilak Swaraj Funds, the National Medical College was established at Mumbai, where Ayurveda was made an obligatory part of the curriculum. In the post-independence era also, Ayurvedic colleges had the integrative courses. When Rustom Jal Vakil confirmed (1949) anti-hypertensive activity of *Rauwolfia serpentina* based on the earlier findings of Gananath Sen, Kartick Chandra Bose, and RN Chopra between 1931 and 1933,[44] the world woke up to the potential of Ayurveda.[45] Reserpine, the active principle of the plant, as a depletory of biogenic amines opened up a watershed of new drugs for depression, Parkinson's disease, galactorrhea, etc.

Visionaries such as KN Udupa, Vice Chancellor of Banaras Hindu University (BHU); PJ Deshpande of BHU; and RN Chopra, Director of Regional Research Laboratories, Jammu also adopted integrative approach to bring the BM and TIM systems together for patient's welfare. Later, GV Satyavati, Director General of ICMR; Ranjit Roy Chaudhury, then Chairman of Expert Committee to Formulate Policy and Guidelines for Approval of New Drugs, Clinical Trials and Banning of Drugs; MS Valiathan, National Professor, Government of India; Ashok Vaidya, Research Director, Medical Research Centre, Kasturba Health Society; Sharadini Dahanukar, Professor and Head, Department of Pharmacology, Seth GS Medical College and KEM Hospital; and several others have promoted the integrative approach for research on traditional remedies. Presently, Bhushan Patwardhan as National Research Professor of AYUSH is overseeing the research activities for the Ministry of AYUSH. Gujarat Ayurved University, Jamnagar, upscaled in 2020 as Institute of Teaching and Research in Ayurveda (ITRA) is a leading institution among others to use this integrative medicine (IM) approach. This is now being followed in other leading Ayurveda institutions including National Institute of Ayurveda, Jaipur (upscaled to Deemed University). The TDU, Bengaluru has also contributed significantly to IM. Their Journal of Ayurveda and Integrated Medicine has provided a well-indexed platform for such research papers.

It is to be noted that it was only much later in 1994, that Andrew Weil from the University of Arizona, US initiated IM.[46] As stated earlier the National Health Policies of the Ministry of Health and Family Welfare have recommended mainstreaming of AYUSH with BM.[47] In fact, IM is the emerging strategy for close collaboration between system-partners for patient-centric treatment to reduce morbidity and mortality of chronic and unresolvable disease conditions. The WHO recognizes this as an important strategy. Recognizing IM's importance, NCCAM (National Center for Complementary and Alternative Medicine), a NIH (National Institutes of Health) institute in USA, converted its name to NCCIH (National Center for Complementary and Integrative Health). Several academic centers in US, EU countries, Africa, Latin America, and Asian countries have launched IM initiative. Presently, integration of ASU drugs and Yoga with BM are being tried across the country by Research Councils under the Ministry of AYUSH and some private institutes in an attempt to improve health care and generate scientific evidence. There have been some notable achievements through such integration in filariasis in Kasargod, Kerala,[48] and rheumatoid arthritis in Coimbatore, Tamil Nadu.[49] The approaches of reverse pharmacology, ayurgenomics, system biology tools, and systematic reviews can provide useful and hopeful insights and new hypotheses for TIM research in future.

Many challenges/issues have been identified in TIM research and many lessons learnt in the process to enable acceptable evidence. The main areas of research issues in TIM pertain to chemical-manufacturing-control (CMC), nonclinical studies, clinical trials, and ethical dimensions.[50]

CHEMICAL-MANUFACTURING-CONTROL

All stages of drug development involve CMC, which is related to quality of the product starting from collection of the plant, identifying it and then developing the product. The potency of a plant depends on the source, time of collection, season, and soil. These are described in the authoritative texts as standards for preparing the appropriate formulation. Pharmacognosy identifies the specific plant and differentiates it from adulterants. There should not be any contamination with pesticides, herbicides, fungus, microbials, toxins, and heavy metals.

Traditional Indian medicines cannot be subjected to the same rigor used for specific chemical quality of synthetic drugs, as most of these are complex combinations and their crude extract having uncharacterized constituents, which may not show the side effects of the active ingredient, e.g., *Sarpagandha (Rauwolfia serpentina)*. TIM drugs, with proper range of concentration of the ingredients have successfully shown safety and efficacy in clinical trials. Chemical fingerprinting identifies markers, some of which may be bioactive and help in checking batch-to-batch variation of manufactured product. Since traditional remedies usually have short shelf life, increasing their stability and shelf life and controlling their batch-to-batch variation could be a challenging task, when used for research. Therefore, for research purpose, it would be desirable to prepare the formulation expected to have short shelf-life in bulk amount to avoid this variation. Phytopharmaceuticals are purified and standardized fractions developed from medicinal plant or its parts having minimum four bioactive ingredients and this is treated as new drug as per the New Drugs and Clinical Trial Rules, 2019.[51]

An adequate literature survey for better identification of drug and an easier access to source for collection of the ingredients is desirable. Sometimes use of a common name for different plants could be confusing, e.g., *Brahmi,* an Indian name, is used for both *Bacopa monnieri* and *Centella asiatica* in different geographical locations. The traditional medicine Section at Uppsala Center in Sweden is attempting to have a botanically harmonized listing of plants from different parts of the world. Therefore, it is clear that a good botanist, preferably a taxonomist, identifies the plant as the first step toward standardization because the part taken should be authentic and of prescribed age. Information about each plant ingredient must be collected, authenticated, and maintained, as voucher specimens and appropriate SOPs should also be in place for standardization. It is necessary to have a repository of pharmacopoeial reference standards for procuring raw drug material for R&D and manufacture of ASU drugs or other herbals. As per the Convention of Biodiversity, it is desirable to maintain a repository of genetic resources of plants. Ministry of AYUSH is setting up a regional raw drug repository at the National Institute of Siddha in collaboration with the Regional Research Institute of Unani Medicine (RRIUM) and Siddha Central Research Institute (SCRI), with all being located at Chennai.

There is also an urgent need to find alternative synthetic and semisynthetic analogs of the derivatives of the plant drugs from dwindling natural source to sustain the ever-increasing demand of such products across the globe. This calls for greater investment in building capacity in the related scientific fields and cultivation on a large scale of at least the perennial and annual medicinal plants. More and more public–private partnerships will be required for this purpose. The National Medicinal Plants Board has to be strengthened with greater resources and personnel and the Forest Department also should be on a constant vigil to prevent denudation of our biodiversity rich forests because of wild scavenging. The tribal or rural folk should be made partners and beneficiaries in the conservation programs for salvaging the trees/herbs. It should also strictly implement replanting of medicinal plants in the forests during the appropriate seasons. Preventing exploitation of plant resources, developing techniques such as tissue culture and hydroponics, and undertaking networking to share resources and capacities would be the ideal order of the day.

Rule 158 (B) in the Drugs and Cosmetics Rules, 1945 provides for "guidelines for issue of license with respect to the Ayurveda, Siddha, or Unani drugs" for their commercial usage.[52] Considering the high demand for quality drugs, more academia–industry collaboration is solicited to augment and upgrade the testing and manufacturing of standardized ASU preparations at reasonable rates. The manufacturers can use government service laboratories for identification, standardization, and establishment of purity of the raw materials for abiding by GMP requirements. It should be noted that the classical texts do describe the quality requirements. This was evidenced when medicated thread *Kshaarasootra* was prepared as per the requirements described in the *Sushruta Samhita* by the ICMR's Centre of Advanced Research at the Regional Research Laboratories, Jammu for research on anal fistula. It may be noted that the DCA has a provision to waive off the requirement of manufacturing license for Vaidyas and Hakims who prepare medicines for dispensing to their patients alone and the access to which is all the more convenient for the rural folk for their health care.

Drugs derived from genetically modified plants through recombinant deoxyribonucleic acid (rDNA) technologies need to be processed as per existing guidelines and regulatory procedures for genetically modified organisms (GMOs)—the Environment Protection Act (EPA) 1986 and the rDNA safety guidelines and regulations 1990/1994 and revised guidelines for research in transgenic plants,1998 of the DBT.

NONCLINICAL STUDIES

In addition to the homoeopathic drugs, the plant-based drugs are divided into phytopharmaceuticals, ASU drugs, and patent and proprietary drugs. Crude extract (aqueous or aqueous-alcoholic extracts) or active pharmaceutical ingredient can be isolated from the herbs for drug development. In consultation with the Central Councils of Research under the Department of Indian systems of Medicine and Homoeopathy/Department of AYUSH (named so respectively then), ICMR had indicated in its Ethical Guidelines of 2000 and 2006, that for those formulations which have to be used for >3 months or there is toxicity reported in the literature or if large-scale phase III clinical trials have to be conducted, then limited toxicity studies in two species of animals for a period of 4–6 weeks are required. Subsequently, the safety/toxicity guidelines to evaluate plant-based drugs as per Guidelines of Organization for Economic Co-operation and Development (OECD) have been published by the Central Council for Research in Ayurvedic Sciences (CCRAS) in 2018.[34] The phytochemical constituents of a herbal drug can together target multi-tissues or organs to maintain a balance for beneficial activity in a particular ailment. The precise phytochemical constituents as bioactive molecules for pharmacokinetics and bioavailability studies on single herbs are easier to identify than in the case of polyherbal formulations (PHFs) due to complex interactive constituents. System biology approach may be a more useful methodology to assess the holistic effect. Mechanism of action studies may provide evidence at molecular level but the ideal models to be used for such studies are also not so easy to determine.

CLINICAL STUDIES

Widely used TIM drugs can be validated for safety and effectiveness by big data studies in Ayurvedic pharmacoepidemiolgy and multicentric observational studies with objective markers. Even repositioning of TIM drugs, for new indications, can follow these approaches.

Designing RCTs for efficacy of a traditional medicine as a holistic trial design tailored to an individual's constitution and host-disease variability could be challenging. Several reporting guidelines indirectly provide guidance for proper designing of study. For epidemiological observational studies STROBE (Strengthening the Reporting of Observational Studies in Epidemiology) Guidelines, 2007, and for reporting of case reports CARE Guidelines (CAse REports), 2013, can be used. Consolidated Standards of Reporting Trials (CONSORT) for herbal medical interventions could be a guiding framework to prepare well-designed RCTs.[53] SPIRIT (Standard Protocol Items: Recommendations for Interventional Trials), 2013 statement can also be adopted to design clinical trial protocols. Although RCTs, especially the double-blinded ones are the accepted standard of clinical research, it may not always provide the answer for efficacy, which is otherwise well documented in the classical texts and clinical experience.[54] Also, for certain interventions double-blinded approach may not be possible, e.g., medicated thread (*Kshaarasootra*) versus surgical intervention for anal fistula. In RCT using herbals with placebo control, it is sometimes difficult to have color, smell, and taste-matched placebo. Sometimes partial randomization patient preference trial is also used where patient is allowed to choose preferred treatment.[55] In single subject (participant) clinical trial or *N* of 1, the outcome of different interventions related to a particular complaint in same patient is studied. The objective of such a study using data driven criteria is to find optimal or best intervention and least side-effects, if any, in the patient.[56] There is a great need to explore sequential trial designs after $n = 1$ study. Nevertheless, limitation of such a study is that it cannot be extrapolated to larger numbers of patients. Sometimes careful and well-monitored observational studies[57] may provide valuable information on the doses to be used to suit the patient's constitution and relevant side effects/rare AEs, especially the drug-herb interaction. NCCIH recognizes that 10-15 years of anecdotal clinical experience is sufficient to allow conduct of clinical trials in the reverse pharmacology mode, which has three stages—(1) experiential, (2) exploratory, and (3) experimental. Based on types of outcome expected, single case design, black box design, stepped wedge design, ethnographic study, quality of life (QoL) studies, and qualitative studies can be carried out. When experimenting a new treatment, pilot studies may be undertaken first. The newer methodologies are Adaptive trials, Umbrella, and Basket trials having biomarker/genetic basis for response, and in the wake of COVID-19 pandemic, the platform trials, e.g., RECOVERY trial of UK. As far as possible, the principles and the concomitant nondrug modalities of treatment of traditional medicine systems should be retained.

Very often statistical analysis may fail to prove the actual positive effect of TIM intervention. As Tröhler points out,[58] the methods used have to facilitate interpretation of the sum results of "arithmetic observationalists and experimentalists". Adaptive designs where methodological and statistical modifications can be done during the period of trial may serve as a better option. Analytic methodology will also have to address the multiple dimensions of the treatment outcomes in terms of response of body, mind, and genetic make-up. In placebo-controlled RCTs, analysis of outcome should factor the placebo effect.

Phytopharmaceuticals need to undergo the steps required for new drugs while ASU drugs for traditional indication applied to matching BM conditions can use reverse pharmacology approach to validate the claim. A multi-disciplinary approach involving good collaboration between TIM and BM practitioners as a team, works well for the scientific conduct of research using traditional medicines for scientific validation of efficacy of TIM. It is essential to provide sufficient information on safety and efficacy if the public and healthcare providers are to make informed decisions on the use of traditional medicine. Unfortunately, BM practitioner researchers cannot prescribe medicines which are proven to be safe and efficacious by them in association with the TIM practitioner researchers due to legal restrictions, as they are not trained in that discipline. At the same time, TIM practitioners are legally allowed to dispense BM medications in some states.

The clinical trials should be conducted following GCP norms and appropriate ethical guidelines as brought out by the Government from time to time but GCP compliant high-quality research required from the research community calls for a sustained financial support from government and industry.

ETHICAL ISSUES

The ICMR National Ethical Guidelines, 2017 are applicable to all researchers while technical details pertaining to research in TIM now fall under the ambit of the Ministry of AYUSH. These guidelines have 12 general principles which apply to all types of human research and concern all stakeholders responsible for good conduct of research **(Box 1)**. These principles are mainly based on the universal principles of respect for persons, beneficence, nonmaleficence, and justice and also the Global Code for Conduct of Research in Resource Poor Settings for collaborative research (GCC).[59] Clause 15 of New Drug and Clinical Trials Rule has indirectly legislated these guidelines. Only specific ethical issues related to TIM research will be mentioned here.

Scientific rationale: The research should address the societal need and potential benefit that may ensue. Scientific review of the research proposal is essential. Any clinical trial that has to be undertaken using modern scientific methodologies should be a collaborative effort between the researchers of TIM and BM as equal partners whether on national or international basis. Clarifications may be sought whether the product has been ensured of not having adulterants and whether prior information on dose finding, toxicity, and herb-drug interaction, if any, has been verified and submitted.

BOX 1: General Ethical Principles (ICMR National Ethical Guidelines, 2017).

1. Essentiality
2. Voluntariness
3. Nonexploitation
4. Social responsibility
5. Privacy and confidentiality
6. Risk minimization
7. Professional competence
8. Maximization of benefit
9. Institutional arrangements
10. Transparency and accountability
11. Totality of responsibility
12. Environment protection

Benefit-risk assessment: Any proposal should be evaluated for the probability and magnitude of risk/harm that a participant may be subjected to—less than minimal risk, minimal risk, minor risk over minimal risk or low risk and more than minimal risk or high risk. Depending on the type of risk, the EC would determine whether the proposal would be exempted from review or undergo expedited or full committee review. Safety reports should be sent on timely basis and EC should address the issue as per the guidelines/regulations.

Design: To get the generalizable knowledge, the design of the study should be duly reviewed by EC to ensure whether the research is feasible and protects rights, safety, and well-being of the participants in that setting. Since ECs of BM institutions usually do not have the expertise to review such proposals, an appropriate TIM expert should be co-opted or asked to review the proposal and to provide comments. The different designs feasible for TIM studies that can be adopted are described earlier. Placebo in controlled trials should be chosen only if there is no other alternative standard of care. After the trial is over, it is ethically required that the participants in placebo arm are taken care of, by giving the test medication for a reasonable period or alternative as the case may be, if the trial shows it to be beneficial and feasible to do so.

Informed consent: Informed consent document should make it very clear to the participants, the treatment methodology, especially when placebo and blinding modalities are used. This is particularly important in chronic diseases where participants prefer TIM to BM. Compensation for participation and injury during the research period should be addressed in every proposal including the informed consent document. Care should be taken to prevent therapeutic misconception.

Collaborative or interdisciplinary: The local practices should be respected. BM researchers cannot conduct a trial based only on a survey of ancient literature or classical texts. They have to partner with the TIM researcher. It would be ideal to have a multidisciplinary expert group to guide the designing of the study and its evaluation.

Intellectual property rights (IPR): If there is possibility of potential commercialization, then there should be benefit sharing, especially if the knowledge has come from a community. The wrong patenting of Indian plants as wound healers—US patent on *Curcuma longa* (turmeric) and the European patent on *Azadirachta indica* (Neem)—resulted in creating Traditional Knowledge Digital Library (TKDL) as a defensive step to maintain a database on medicinal plants described in the authoritative textbooks of First Schedule of DCA. To prevent biopiracy, this database has been made accessible to several patent offices across the globe through a nondisclosure agreement. But unfortunately, TKDL has thwarted the R&D on Ayurvedic plants for IPR on products, due to declaration of prior art. This information should be made available to R&D institutions and pharma research centers of the country to guide better research and improve quality of manufacture of TIM formulations. In a biodiversity rich country like India, the untapped tribal knowledge of ethnomedicine can be subjected to commercialization by patenting the practice or herbal-based drug molecules. Prior informed consent to protect the rights of the owner of the knowledge, as well as access and benefit sharing, are to be discussed prior to initiating research in such cases. In fact, India has set an example by providing for the first time in the world, with a 50% share in the commercial gains to a tribal community (*Kani*) in Kerala,[59,60] in return for its knowledge about a medicinal plant *Trichopus zeylanicus* (Arogyappacha or "Jeevani") from which an antistress and antifatigue drug was prepared and commercialized. It would be the ethical responsibility of the researcher/research team to work out mechanisms for utilizing appropriately the returns for the welfare of such communities.

Training: Training in research methodology, GCP, and GMPs adapted to the needs of the systems are required. ASU-GCP should be updated regularly and followed for all the TIM clinical research in the country. For the farming sector engaged in cultivation of medicinal plants, training in good agriculture practices, good harvesting practices, and good collection practices are also required to give best yields.

CONCLUSION

India has a unique pluralistic healthcare system. Recognizing the strengths and limitations of both the BM and TIM is important, as these can be utilized appropriately as an interdisciplinary approach in the best interest of the patients. The continuum of AYUSH systems, an immensely rich biodiversity, a robust biomedical research base, vast clinical material and a growing global interest in natural drugs inspire suitable growth in TIM research and integrative perspective in medicine. The latter requires a development chain of quality and standard operative procedures. The spectrum covers good agricultural practice, good transport/storage, good botanical/pharmaceutical standardization, good laboratory practice, good ethical/clinical practice, and good regulatory mandates. There is also a need for expert monitoring of these practices, adequate documentation, and meticulous analyses at all the levels.

The rampant damage likely to be caused to the environment due to large-scale harvesting of natural materials need to be timely addressed in order to preserve the biodiversity. Cultivation of medicinal plants of high demand, is the easiest modality to be implemented urgently. Maintenance of standards and quality control of traditional formulations should be tackled by increasing the number of trained personnel and well-equipped analytical laboratories. For these to actualize, we need to have frequent training programs in reverse pharmacology, research methodologies, biostatistics, ethics, GCP and any other relevant areas. Much more needs to be done to safeguard the nation's heritage of traditional medical systems and promote innovations through integrative research and knowledge protection.

The safety and efficacy studies of herbal or herbo-mineral formulations should be conducted by adhering to relevant ethical and regulatory guidelines. Suitable incorporation of regulatory provisions regarding clinical trials of TIM in the DCA and mandatory regulatory approval for such trials is poised to lead the way to the conduct of robust studies. Accreditation of ECs dealing with TIM proposals by suitable regulatory authority will ensure the credibility of studies being conducted. Registration of all clinical trials with the Clinical Trial Registry of India (CTRI) will help in disseminating the information to all stakeholders in research and save duplication of research efforts.

The "One Nation–One Healthcare" proposed by the NITI Aayog is a futuristic vision to utilize the traditional wisdom to improve the health care and economy of India through interdisciplinary approach. That will make India a world leader in health care by designing scientifically valid and ethically conducted clinical trials on traditional formulations, for global acceptance of standardized interventions, which are safe and efficacious.

ACKNOWLEDGMENT

Dr N Srikanth, Deputy Director General, Central Council for Research in Ayurvedic Sciences (CCRAS), New Delhi, India.

Disclaimer: The views expressed in the document by Dr Pradeep Dua are solely his and may not be construed as the views of BIS/CCRAS/Ministry of AYUSH.

REFERENCES

1. Valiathan MS. An Ayurvedic view of life. Curr Sci. 2009; 96(9):1186-92.
2. Patwardhan B. Ayurveda and Systems Biology. Ann Ayurvedic Med. 2014;3(1-2) 5-7.
3. Narayanaswamy V. Origin and development of Ayurveda: (a brief history). Anc Sci Life.1981;1(1):1-7.
4. Valiathan MS. The Legacy of Charaka, 1st edition. Chennai: Orient Longman; 2003. p. xvii.
5. Iwu MM, Gbodossou E. The role of traditional medicine. Lancet. 2000;356 Suppl:S3.
6. World Health Organization. WHO traditional medicine strategy: 2014-2023. Geneva: World Health Organization; 2013.
7. Vaidya ADB. Reverse pharmacological correlates of Ayurvedic drug actions. Indian J Pharmacol. 2006;38:311-5.
8. Patwardhan B, Vaidya ADB, Chorghade M, Joshi SP. Reverse pharmacology and systems approaches for drug discovery and development. Curr Bioact Compd. 2008;4:201-12.
9. Mukerji M, Prasher B. Ayurgenomics: a new approach in personalized and preventive medicine. Sci Cult. 2011;77: 10-7.
10. Prasher B, Varma B, Kumar A, Khuntia BK, Pandey R, Narang A, et al. Ayurgenomics for stratified medicine: TRISUTRA consortium initiative across ethnically and geographically diverse Indian populations. J Ethnopharmacol. 2017;197: 274-93.
11. Patwardhan B, Gangadharan G, Tillu G, Vaidya ADB. Systems Ayurveda: Conceptual foundation and logic. Conference at FRLHT, Bengaluru; 2012. DOI: 10.13140/RG2.2.13792.30722.
12. Vaidya A, Roy A, Chaguturu, R. How to rekindle drug discovery process through integrative therapeutic targeting? Expert Opin Drug Discov. 2018;13:893-8.
13. World Health Organization. Traditional Medicine Strategy 2002–2005. Geneva: World Health Organization; 2002.
14. World Health Organization. WHO Global Health Report on Traditional and Complementary Medicine 2019. Geneva: World Health Organization; 2019.
15. Ministry of AYUSH. National Health Policy on Indian Systems of Medicine and Homeopathy. New Delhi, Government of India: Ministry of AYUSH; 2017.
16. Witt C, Brinkhaus B, Willich SN. Future medical doctors need to be informed about CAM to ensure safe and competent patient care. GMS Z Med Ausbild. 2010;27(2):Doc22.
17. Cant S. Medical Pluralism, Mainstream Marginality or Subaltern Therapeutics? Globalisation and the Integration of 'Asian' Medicines and Biomedicine in the UK. Soc Cult South Asia. 2020;6(1):31-51.
18. Editorial. Complementary Medicine: time for critical engagement. Lancet. 2000;356(9247):2023.
19. National Center for Complementary and Integrative Health. Congressional Justification FY 2021. [online] Available from: https://www.nccih.nih.gov/about/budget/congressional/fy2021.
20. Government of India. Ministry of AYUSH. [online] Available from: https://health.ncog.gov.in/login.
21. Kumar NK. Informed consent: Past and present. Perspect Clin Res. 2013;4(1):21-5.
22. Kantoori GH. The legacy of Hippocrates and other ancient physicians and learned scholars of this system of Medicine. Kamilussanah, 1st edition. New Delhi: Idara Kitab ul Shifa; 2010. pp. 10-11.
23. Shastri A. Ashmari Chikitsa. Sushruta Samhita Chikitsa Sthana, 6th edition. Varanasi, Uttar Pradesh: Chaukhamba Sanskrit Samsthana; 1987. p. 42.
24. Shukla V, Tripathi R. Chikitsa Sthana. Caraka Samhita. Delhi: Chaukhamba Sanskrit Pratishthan; 2007. p. 314.
25. Valiathan MS. Bioethics and Ayurveda. Indian J Med Ethics. 2008;5(1):29-30.
26. Saper RB, Kales SN, Paquin J, Burns MJ, Eisenberg DM, Davis RB, et al. Heavy metal content of ayurvedic herbal medicine products. JAMA. 2004;292(23):2868-3.
27. Inter System Biomedica Ethics Committee. [online] Available from: www.isbec.org [Last accessed October, 2021].
28. Indian Council of Medical Research. Policy Statement on Ethical Considerations Involved in Research on Human Subjects. New Delhi: Indian Council of Medical Research; 1980.

29. Pandya SK. Organizing a public debate: Ethical guidelines on biomedical research in humans. Nat Med J India. 1998;11:204-6.
30. Indian Council of Medical Research. Ethical Guidelines for Biomedical research on Human Subjects. New Delhi: Indian Council of Medical Research; 2000.
31. Indian Council of Medical Research. Ethical Guidelines for Biomedical research on Human Participants. New Delhi: Indian Council of Medical Research; 2006.
32. Indian Council of Medical Research. National Ethical Guidelines for Biomedical and Health Research involving Human Participants. New Delhi: Indian Council of Medical Research; 2017.
33. Ministry of AYUSH, Central Council for Research in Ayurvedic Sciences (2021). General Guidelines for Drug Development of Ayurvedic Formulations. [online] Available from: http://www.ccras.nic.in/content/general-guideline-series [Last accessed October, 2021].
34. Ministry of AYUSH, Central Council for Research in Ayurvedic Sciences (2021). General Guidelines of Safety/Toxicity Evaluation of Ayurvedic Formulations. [online] Available from: http://www.ccras.nic.in/content/general-guideline-series [Last accessed October, 2021].
35. Ministry of AYUSH, Central Council for Research in Ayurvedic Sciences. (2021). General Guidelines for Clinical Evaluation of Ayurvedic Interventions. [online] Available from: http://www.ccras.nic.in/content/general-guideline-series [Last accessed October, 2021].
36. Ministry of Health and Family Welfare, Central Drugs Standard Control Organization. The Drugs and Cosmetics Act, 1940 and Drugs and Cosmetics Rules, 1945. New Delhi: Ministry of Health and Family Welfare; 1940.
37. Kumar NK, Dua PK. Status of regulation on traditional medicine formulations and natural products: Whither is India? Curr Sci. 2016;25:293-301.
38. Nandini KK, Muthuswamy V, Ganguly NK. Initiatives of Indian Council of Medical Research in scientific validation of traditional medicine. In: Ayurveda and its Scientific Aspects. New Delhi: Joint Publication of Department of Ayurveda, Yoga, Unani Siddha and Homeopathy, and Council for Scientific and Industrial Research; 2006.
39. Satyavati GV. Research on Indian Medicinal Plants: In Indian Council of Medical Research Bulletin. 1972;2(4)
40. Vaidya RA, Aloorkar SD, Sheth AR, Pandya SK. Activity of bromoergocriptine, Mucuna pruriens and L-dopa in the control of hyperprolactinaemia. Neurol India. 1978;26:179-82.
41. Mashelkar RA. Foreword in Integrative perspectives. Bhatt N (Ed). Mumbai: IASTAM; 2020.
42. Patwardhan B, Vaidya AB. Natural products drug discovery: accelerating the clinical candidate development using reverse pharmacology approaches. Indian J Exp Biol. 2010;48:220-7.
43. Baghel MS. [online] Available from: https://ayurveda-healthcare.info/content/ayurveda-research-database-ard [Last accessed October 2021].
44. Roy P. Global pharma and local science: The untold tale of reserpine. Indian J Psychiatry. 2018;60(Suppl 2):S277-S283.
45. Jain S, Murthy P. The other Bose: an account of missed opportunities in the history of neurobiology in India. Curr Sci. 2000;97:266-9.
46. Melchart D. From Complementary to integrative medicine and Health: do we need a change in nomenclature? Complement Med Res. 2018;25:76-8.
47. Katoch D, Sharma JS, Banerjee S, Biswas R, Das B, Goswami D, et al. Government policies and initiatives for development of Ayurveda. J Ethnopharmacol. 2017;197(2):25-31.
48. Narahari SR, Ryan TJ, Bose KS, Prasanna KS, Aggithaya GM. Integrating modern dermatology and Ayurveda in the treatment of vitiligo and lymphedema in India. Int J Dermatol. 2011;50:310-34.
49. Furst DE, Venkatraman MM, Krishna Swamy BG, McGann M, Booth-Laforce C, Ram Manohar P, et al. Well controlled, double-blind, placebo-controlled trials of classical Ayurvedic treatment are possible in rheumatoid arthritis. Ann Rheum Dis. 2011;70(2):392-3.
50. WHO. Operational guidance: information needed to support clinical trials of herbal products. Geneva: World Health Organization; 2005.
51. Ministry of Health & Family Welfare, Central Drugs Standard Control Organization. New Drugs and Clinical Trial Rules. New Delhi: Ministry of Health & Family Welfare; 2019.
52. Ministry of Health and Family Welfare, Central Drugs Standard Control Organization. Drugs and Cosmetics Act, 1940. New Delhi: Ministry of Health & Family Welfare; 1940.
53. Sikorskii A, Wyatt G, Victorson D, Faulkner G, Rahbar MH. Methodological issues in trials of complementary and alternative medicine interventions. Nurs Res. 2009;58(6):444-51.
54. Richardson J. The use of randomized control trials in complementary therapies: exploring the Issues. J Adv Nurs. 2000;32:398-406.
55. Wasmann KA, Wijsman P, van Dieren S, Bemelman W, Buskens C. Partially randomised patient preference trials as an alternative design to randomised controlled trials: systematic review and meta-analyses. BMJ open. 2019;9(10):e031151.
56. Lillie EO, Patay B, Diamant J, Issell B, Topol EJ, Schork NJ. The n-of-1 clinical trial: the ultimate strategy for individualizing medicine? Per Med. 2011;8(2):161-73.
57. Patwardhan B, Mashelkar RA. Traditional medicine-inspired approaches to drug discovery: Can Ayurveda show the way forward? Drug Discov Today. 2009;14:804-11.
58. Tröhler U. To Improve the Evidence of Medicine: the 18th Century British Origins of a Critical Approach. J R Soc Med. 2001;94(4):204-5.
59. TRUST Consortium (2018). Global Code of Conduct for Research in Resource-Poor Settings. [online] Available from: https://www.globalcodeofconduct.org [Last accessed October, 2021].
60. World Intellectual Property Organization (2020). Using Traditional Knowledge to Revive the Body and a Community. [online] Available from: https://www.wipo.int/ipadvantage/en/details.jsp?id=2599 [Last accessed October, 2021].

CHAPTER 9

Ethical Considerations in Organ and Tissue Transplantation

Tulika Seth, Sujata Mohanty

ABSTRACT

Current clinical practices for organ transplant and hematopoietic stem cell transplant (HSCT), also known as bone marrow transplant, are well established and the ethics, rules, and regulatory issues have been well documented. The lifesaving procedure of HSCT with well-established, altruistic volunteer registries maintaining anonymity of unrelated donors are the norm in many countries. These have also been started in India to benefit patients who do not have a matched related donor. Ethical issues around related minors as donors and ensuring awareness of costs and outcomes in alternative donor transplantation such as matched, mismatched, unrelated transplant, or haplo-transplant must be discussed with the families to ensure informed decision before giving consent. All transplants carry a risk of complications including mortality. These factors depend on patient characteristics as well as the type of transplant. Most countries have laws for nonrenewable tissue and organ transplant to prevent trafficking and protect poor donors from being coerced into donation. Deceased (previously called cadaver) organ programs need to ensure equitable organ allocation, to ensure benefit to needy and sick patients. Most altruistic family donations do not cause major problems, because the patients are counseled for lifelong immunosuppression and increased risks of infections and malignancy. This chapter elaborates on the accepted transplantation procedures for all types of organ and tissue transplants and related ethical issues confronted by the donors, recipients, and treating doctors.

HEMATOPOIETIC STEM CELL TRANSPLANTATION

Studies on hematopoiesis have revealed that blood cells have a limited life span, e.g., red blood cells survive only for 120 days. The specialized cells called hematopoietic stem cells (HSCs), residing in the bone marrow differentiate into different kinds of blood cells and are responsible for the continuous supply of blood cells, as they can be cultured in the laboratory and can be transplanted into a compatible host. The first HSCT was performed in 1968, using bone marrow as a source of HSCs. E Donnall Thomas and Joseph E Murray were awarded the Nobel Prize for research in transplant immunology in 1990. JE Murray used radiation and immunosuppression to prevent rejection of transplanted kidneys in twins while the work of ED Thomas showed that HSCs could repopulate in another host when used with appropriate immunosuppression and conditioning regimens. This potential has been used for HSCTs as standard of care for most high-risk acute leukemias, and many relapsed lymphomas, aplastic anemia, hemoglobinopathies, some cancers, hematological and genetic diseases/conditions due to deficient enzymes/substrates, etc. Immune modulation supported by transplantation has now opened new avenues in the treatment of autoimmune diseases and multiple sclerosis. *Hematopoietic stem cell transplants should not be confused with the novel stem cell therapy and research, which is a separate topic by itself.* When HSCT started in the 1970s, there was a high risk of complications and mortality, as the understanding of transplant immunology and human leukocyte antigen (HLA) barriers was still in its early stages. Over the years, careful clinical practice and advancements in the laboratory understanding of HLA system, immunology of graft versus host disease (GVHD), and immune reconstitution have led to better outcomes, safer and more effective conditioning regimens. It has also allowed transplant with donors beyond the syngeneic twin or 100% matched sibling donors, thus enabling many more patients to receive lifesaving HSCT.

The stem cell sources used for HSCT are bone marrow and peripheral blood stem cells (PBSCs) as well as umbilical cord blood (UCB). Hematopoietic stem cell transplant is now a well-accepted therapeutic modality. There are many centers in India, which perform HSCT. However, there are still a number of moral and social questions, which pose problems for transplant physicians and the families of patients.

Types of Hematopoietic Stem Cell Source

Bone Marrow

The HSCs in the bone marrow form blood, and a healthy adult can donate 1,000–1,500 mL of bone marrow without any complications. In order to collect it, the donor needs general anesthesia and prior to this, a complete health evaluation.[1] The general precautions are similar to the guidelines for a blood donor. Risk of general anesthesia is the same as for any major surgery. Pre-existing comorbid conditions need to be evaluated to assess risk for bone marrow harvesting. The long-term data has shown that this is safe in healthy donors.

Peripheral Blood Stem Cells

These are the HSCs from the bone marrow, which are brought into blood circulation. The numbers of circulating HSCs (CD34+) can be increased in peripheral blood by giving a granulocyte-colony stimulating factor (G-CSF). Then these cells can be collected without any need for surgery by peripheral blood apheresis, similar to that done for collecting apheresis platelet concentrates. Initially, PBSCs were only being used for auto and related allogeneic transplants, but now their use is becoming more common for unrelated HLA-matched donors too, who are also given G-CSF. The use of G-CSF is associated with mild to moderate bone pain, relieved with paracetamol. Only 9% stated the pain was severe and 1% considered the pain "intolerable" when unrelated donors were followed for 4 years post donation without any adverse effects.[2] Thromboembolic side effects of G-CSF were reported in patients of multiple myeloma, lymphomas, etc. undergoing autologous PBSCs collection for autotransplant.[3] These include pulmonary embolism, deep vein thrombosis, and asymptomatic catheter-related thrombosis (approximately 1%).[3] In a large study from Europe looking at both related and unrelated donors, five fatalities were detected in related male donors who were of older age.[4] This was a retrospective study and exact causality to bone marrow or PBSC donation was not identified in all cases, though one was linked to pulmonary embolism.[4] Hence care and a thorough examination of the donor is necessary. No physicians should coerce a donor and the donation needs to be made after free voluntary informed consent. Proper psychological and medical evaluation of the donor is required. A decision should be made only after complete informed deliberations. If the unrelated donor does not agree to take G-CSF, bone marrow may be collected instead. There is very little risk of donation, as bone marrow is renewed like blood. Long-term studies have shown that the persons who donated either bone marrow or PBSCs are without permanent side effects.[1,2] Umbilical cord blood can also be a source of stem cells, but the volume makes it sufficient only for pediatric patients. More discussion on this is given in the following sections of Umbilical Cord Blood Transplant and Special Ethical Considerations in Cord Blood Banking.

Type of Donors

Human Leukocyte Antigen-matched Sibling

Hematopoietic stem cell transplantation from HLA-matched donors produce the best results; HLA-matched siblings are the ideal donors of HSCs.

Human Leukocyte Antigen-matched Unrelated Donor

If a matched sibling donor is unavailable then an unrelated and fully HLA-matched donor is the next best choice. Unrelated donors should donate only with altruistic motives and no compensation should be given. There are several international donor registries with millions of donors. Most Indian transplant centers were till now getting HLA-matched HSC from these donor registries, namely, National Marrow Donor Program (NMDP) (USA), German National Registry of Blood Stem Cell Donors (DKMS), Anthony Nolan (UK), etc. Unrelated transplants are standard of care for many diseases and are safe both for the patient and the donor.[5] The risk of donor attrition after matching and the risk of GVHD are higher in unrelated transplants.[5]

Haplo (half)-identical Family Donor

If a fully HLA-matched donor is unavailable then 1–2 mismatched donors or even haploidentical family donors may be acceptable in some situations. This depends on many factors such as extent of mismatch, the disease of the patient, and other clinical information.[5]

Umbilical cord blood can be from an HLA-matched sibling or from a public cord blood bank which can provide unrelated UCB for transplantation.

The degree of acceptable donor disparity depends on the disease and urgency for transplant. The transplant doctor and the treating team can decide this best.[5] There have been legal issues related to unrelated haplo-transplant in India when the outcome of transplant was adverse. The major ethical concerns revolve around informed consent for these procedures, due to the cost and toxicity. Adequate counseling about risks is required.

Except for few government hospitals in India performing these procedures free of cost and some state governments providing insurance to those below the poverty line, HSCTs are expensive procedures, which some government/insurance company refuse to pay, with only a few government hospitals in India performing these procedures at present. Therefore, the cost is often borne by the family. If the family is not well informed of the risk of mortality, or have paid with the hope of cure, they will feel despair and anger if a fatal outcome occurs after so much time, money, and efforts put in. However, no doctors can guarantee positive results in any individual case.

Ethical Issues in Relation to Patient and Donor in Hematopoietic Stem Cell Transplant

Attrition

Attrition is when a person volunteers to donate her/his bone marrow and allows the preliminary HLA (blood) test reports to be put in the database, but when requested for a sample for confirmatory typing or at any other point pertaining to HSC donation, drops out. There are over 50 donor registries with >18.5 million registered donors across the globe, yet with very few Indians. Donor attrition is an issue in ethnic donors even in the international registries.[6,7]

Donor Consent

If the donors or the recipients are minors, then the question of autonomy and consent arises. Can a child make a well-informed decision regarding donation of stem cells? If the parents make this decision, are the parents overstepping the boundaries of their responsibility? This issue of validity of a minor's assent is very difficult to resolve.[8] There should be a combined discussion with the parents, physicians and other members of the transplant team. If the donor child or recipient child is mature enough to understand the implications, they should be included in the decision-making process. This is a gray area since the majority of international and national ethics committees leave this decision to the parent, as it is done with the motive of saving their affected child.[8,9] The procedure of stem cell collection by either bone marrow harvest or from peripheral blood for stem cells is safe and easy to perform. This is a renewable resource and no medical consequence to the minor sibling donors has been reported to date. Hence risks of permanent harm are minimal. With appropriate medical care, this is a very safe procedure, and most physicians feel comfortable allowing siblings to donate HSCs. The type of HSCs to be collected depends on the patient's disease, and to some degree on the donor's weight, or weight difference between patient and donor.

Patient/Recipient Consent

In all transplants including matched related sibling transplant, and to a higher degree in matched unrelated and haploidentical transplants, there is risk of mortality and morbidity, and, patients may be at more risk due to age, disease, prior therapy, or comorbidity.[5,10] The disease for which transplantation is being performed may also have different complications, risks, and outcome, hence patient-specific counseling is necessary. Complications can occur due to conditioning regimen, infections, and GVHD, an immune consequence of HSCT. GVHD is a serious complication, as its acute grade IV can be life-threatening, and chronic GVHD can severely compromise quality of life (QOL). Several scoring systems like hematopoietic cell transplantation-specific comorbidity index (HCT-CI),[10] etc. are used to identify patients at high risk at the pretransplant stage, but these scores do not predict those who may develop grade IV steroid refractory GVHD or serious infections post-transplant. The prevention and prediction of GVHD are not 100%. These complications can occur in all types of allotransplants. Occurrence of GVHD requires additional immunosuppression, which puts the patient at risk for serious and unusual infections. Post-transplant immune reconstitution may take 6 months to many years, depending on the type of transplant and GVHD status. In our experience, counseling patients who have refractory or high risk underlying disease or multiple comorbidities which puts them at high risk of death from the HSCT and low risk of success, requires time and care. Even when only a 10% chance of success is stated, this is taken in an extremely positive context. Due to the emotional involvement, and the urge to try a lifesaving treatment, families ignore the fact that there is a 90% chance of failure.[11] Hence several meetings are required to ensure understanding before informed consent is obtained and all issues discussed need to be documented.

Psychological Impact

If the patient dies in the setting of a related transplant, the donor may feel grief, survivor guilt, and anger. Hence, counseling of both the patient and donor is required prior to the transplant procedure.[8,12]

Cost

This is a lifesaving procedure and government assistance programs are available. These are also expensive procedures and require excellent training and facilities. There is however, a high infection risk due to immunosuppressive therapy, neutropenia, central lines or the disease state for which the HSCT is being performed. The patient requires close monitoring for rejection, GVHD, and other complications. The immunosuppressive medications and monitoring tests are expensive. Matched unrelated transplant (MUD) incur higher costs as the testing, screening, collection, and transportation costs are high, which vary among different countries. DKMS, NMDP, and Antony Nolan are a few major organizations, which maintain staff, data bases, etc. to help patients find a suitable match. All this costs money. In most countries, the insurance company or government pays the expense. In the Indian context, who should bear these additional costs, is yet unclear. Some insurance companies are paying the equivalent of a sibling allotransplant, the additional cost of the matched unrelated donor has to be borne by the family.

Special Issues Related to Other Common Types of Hematopoietic Stem Cell Transplant

Haploidentical Transplantation

Only 25–30% of patients will have an HLA-matched sibling donor. If an unrelated HLA-matched donor also cannot be found, then haploidentical or half-matched donor transplant can be performed. This has become possible now with newer transplant regimens which take advantage of the engraftment process and certain medications to reduce the risk of GVHD and allow such transplants to be possible.[5] The advantage of haplo-transplants in the Indian scenario is that usually a family donor is available, it is, however, still more expensive than a matched sibling allotransplant, but less expensive than the MUD transplants.

Many centers in India are routinely performing these transplants along with matched transplants for leukemia, aplastic anemia, etc. They are now considered as clinical options (CO) in many National guidelines in the UK, Europe, etc.[5] Haplo-transplants in diseases such as thalassemia major have shown excellent results in countries like Thailand.[13] However, randomized clinical trials are unlikely to happen anywhere in the world as multiple donors for each patient are unavailable.

However, it is important to note that no type of transplant or other medical procedure is without risk. No doctors can guarantee cure or survival. Many review articles and guidelines discuss the standard of care and CO as therapeutic options.[5] However, clinical trials are important as they add to the body of evidence and lead to progress in the field. It is important to note that guidelines are compiled from clinical evidence, which takes years to collect. Also, guidelines need constant updating as new evidence and improvements in practices emerge.

Umbilical Cord Blood Transplant

This is an alternative source of HSCs. It can be collected from the umbilical cord at the time of delivery. Clamping of the cord close to the umbilicus reduces the amount of blood received by the baby, but can increase the yield of cord blood collection. Although trying to get maximum length of the cord to get the cord blood may not be life-threatening to the baby, one has to be cautious that no harm is faced by the donor child.

There is a concern that the conception of a donor child, after the diagnosis of a serious illness in an older sibling may not be in the best interests of the newborn.[14,15] The child may be conceived only to help the other child and not actually be a desired offspring.[14] If the older sibling does not benefit from the transplant, there may be anger and serious repercussions against the donor child. This is one reason that physicians must never advise the conception of another child as a potential HSC donor as there is only a 25–30% chance of one sibling having HLA matching with the recipient.

In genetic conditions such as thalassemia major, the donor child must either be normal or be only a carrier. A chorionic villus sample (CVS) is required to determine the status of the child. The physician cannot and should not recommend the abortion of a baby who is afflicted with a genetic disorder or is not an HLA match for the patient. That decision is left to the parents although this may cause severe mental anguish to the parents.[14,15]

At the time of birth of a newborn, many metabolic disorders may not be diagnosed especially the late onset disorders. This particular factor has been an argument against cord blood collection, from unrelated donors in particular.[15] This risk is reduced somewhat by taking a detailed history of genetic diseases in the family, but cannot be completely eliminated. Even collecting the child's own cord blood may not be completely safe. A study in infants with leukemia showed that their own cord blood showed the presence of leukemia mutation before they had developed the disease. Autologous (self) cord blood cannot cure genetic diseases in the child, as it will also have the defective genes. Hence most professional bodies discourage storing a child's cord blood for future use.[15,16] For profit private cord blood banks are not recommended in the west, but are popular in India. Autologous cord blood banking is expensive and the chance that the cord blood will be used may be, 1 in 200,000.[16] In the USA and Europe, government funded cord blood banks have been set up and the public is encouraged to donate to them.

Special Ethical Considerations in Cord Blood Banking

Consent is taken from the mother for cord blood collection and storage for later use in unrelated HLA-matched patients. The child from whom the cord blood is obtained, does not have any rights and has no control as to where her/his cells may be used. This is a possible issue, though not challenged as yet. With new regulations on genetic material handling, this may be seen as an infringement of the child's rights to her/his genetic material and an invasion of her/his privacy. Certain genetic diseases, which manifest later in life, may be missed at the time of collection of cord blood. This may result in the recipient developing genetic diseases, inherited from the donor, for which she/he was not previously at risk. If at any time, the donor child develops a requirement for HSCT, the family may try to reclaim the cord blood. This may be a problem for the cord blood bank, as the unit may have been utilized already or promised to another patient. In such instances, the donor child should be provided alternate cord blood from any other donor.

There is a benefit of UCB banking for patients of certain minority ethnic groups, who are not well represented in bone marrow registries, since these mostly comprise Caucasian donors.[16] The time to find a match and cost of collection of unrelated cord blood are both less when compared to

TABLE 1: Summary of ethical concerns related to hematopoietic stem cell transplant and cord blood banking.

Stem cell type	Source	Current and anticipated use	Ethical issues
Hematopoietic stem cells such as bone marrow	Bone marrow from HLA-matched related or unrelated donors, haploidentical transplants (in some indications)	Hematopoietic stem cell transplant for genetic and acquired conditions, such as hemoglobinopathies, aplastic anemia, leukemias, etc.	Minor issues related to minor siblings
Peripheral blood stem cells	G-CSF mobilized peripheral blood by apheresis	Hematopoietic stem cell transplant for genetic and acquired conditions, such as hemoglobinopathies, aplastic anemia, leukemias, etc.	None
Umbilical cord blood	Umbilical cord blood, through private or public donations	Understanding of hematopoiesis and transplant biology. Research on expansion, double cord use for adults and better graft versus disease effect	Autologous cord blood banking is expensive and wasteful. Public cord blood banking benefits society and may be advised
All hematopoietic stem cell transplant (HSCT) • Matched sibling • MUD • Haploidentical transplant • Umbilical cord blood transplant	Any	All	• Poor outcome may be expected, so it is necessary to explain all potential complications and risks. To obtain informed patient and donor/family consent. • To follow standard of care and clinical option (CO) guidelines.

(G-CSF: granulocyte-colony stimulating factor; HLA: human leukocyte antigen; MUD: matched unrelated transplant)

unrelated BM/PBSC donations.[5,16] This is one of the main reasons why cord blood transplants are proving to be popular, especially for critically ill children. Though now with better technology even haplo-transplants can help reduce time for finding a donor **(Table 1)**.

Issues Pertaining to Hematopoietic Stem Cell Transplant Research

Research is needed to improve transplant outcomes, prevent complications, and possibly reduce costs. Many basic biology questions relating to improved donor selection, prediction of rejection and relapse remain unanswered.
- Research to decrease risk to the donor and study of long-term side effects of intervention, e.g., use of growth factors to mobilize HSCs.
- Research to decrease the side effects of drugs, pharmacogenetics, improvement of antirejection medications, and their monitoring should be independent of pressure from the pharmaceutical companies.
- Surveillance and novel ways to combat risk of malignancy and post-transplant infections.
- Clinical trials to improve transplant regimens and develop new regimens for improving results as many subsets of patients do poorly with present day regimens.
- Research on QOL and psychological issues in donor and recipient.
- Research on potential strategies to decrease cost of transplantation, indigenous drugs, avoidance of growth factors, and exploration of other techniques.
- Many countries have national registries to report data. An Indian stem cell transplant registry (ISCTR) maintained by the Indian Society for Blood and Marrow Transplantation (ISBMT) society (https://www.isbmt.org/) has been started by CMC, Vellore, to collect data with an aim to measure overall survival, and later:
    - Long-term consequences of HSCT and adverse effects
    - Report survival outcomes—time from diagnosis, time from transplant, or time from recurrence
    - Mitigation of long-term adverse effects by changes in regimen or intervention
- For pediatric patients with slowly progressive forms of inherited metabolic diseases, controlled trials with sufficient follow-up to evaluate the long-term balance of benefit, adverse events, QOL, etc.
- Research into novel applications—such as tissue engineering, stem cell expansion, and stem cell research.

Autologous Bone Marrow Transplant/Hematopoietic Stem Cells

This procedure takes advantage of the plasticity of stem cells, which are transplanted for repair of ischemic cardiac muscle and various other diseases. Auto stem cells (Auto SC) are collected from the patient and reinfused near the myocardium either directly or after manipulation with differentiating factors in vitro. This Auto SC procedure has been shown to regenerate heart muscles in some cases. There is no ethical objection to using autologous stem cells.

However, efficacy trials are needed before such procedure is ethically allowed in practice, as they may give false hope to patients.

SOLID ORGAN AND TISSUE TRANSPLANTATION

The transplantation of solid organs has many ethical, infrastructural, procedural, and legal issues. The donors of organs and tissues are either living or deceased. There is a gamut of ethical and health problems for the living donors, societal dilemmas, and paucity of sustainable infrastructure. This led to the Transplantation of Human Organs Act (THOA) in 1994 and subsequent amendment in 2011 which paved the way for a new National Organ and Tissue Transplant Organization (NOTTO),[17] a National level organization, under the Directorate General of Health Services, Ministry of Health and Family Welfare, Government of India followed by a National Registry in 2015,[18] which was instrumental in augmenting all outcomes. NOTTO is somewhat similar to the National Transplant Organization of Spain and United Network of Organ Sharing of the USA.

Donor Issues—Cadaver Organ and Tissues

The two main sources of organs for transplantation are deceased (previously called cadaveric) and living-related donors. Here the concept of brain death is important as prescribed in the THOA. A deceased or brainstem donor is a dead individual, who has before death wished her/his organs to be donated. However, donation many times has been refused by the family against the wishes of the donors made before their demise. Legally, organs can be harvested from the deceased, only with the consent of the family members. However, rarely the donation could be the desire of the family. The organ once removed from the body needs to be transplanted within a few hours, in order to preserve function. Hence potential recipients are advised to stay in the city and reach the hospitals as soon as they are called with the availability of a donor organ. Deceased organ donation in India is less than the Western world due to many factors, one of them being widely misunderstood concept of brain death, as it is often considered as coma, which is totally disparate.

Brain Death or Brainstem Death

Brain death occurs when the brainstem, which controls important functions such as breathing and blood pressure, fails. This can occur after stroke due to brain hemorrhage, traumatic head injury, brain tumors, encephalitis, cardiac arrest, etc. The person will still have a heart beat for some time but no spontaneous breathing. So a brain-dead individual requires artificial respiration for oxygenation unlike a patient in coma, who may still be able to breathe spontaneously. The heart is able to beat, if supplied with requisite energy as it has its own battery called a pacemaker. As long as the heart beats, most organs are able to work. However, even the heart will cease after a varying interval of time in a brain-dead person. Once the heart stops beating, all the organs will be damaged due to lack of blood supply. Brain death is an irreversible state. The best results of nonliving donor organ transplants are with brainstem dead donor organs or organs transplanted within a few hours of death. In order to assist physicians and families, the THOA, 1994 was formulated and amended in 2011 and notified in 2014.[17,18]

As per the regulations,[17,18] a panel of experts is required to review and declare brainstem death before certifying that it has occurred. What is constituted by brainstem death is clearly specified in the "THOA, 1994". It consists of all permanent and irreversible cessation of functions of the brainstem. The criteria to diagnose brainstem death include the absence of brainstem reflexes tested at least twice with an interval of 6 hours between the two evaluations. Any reversible causes for brainstem dysfunction such as hypothermia, metabolic derangements, and drug intoxication must be excluded.[17,18] After the panel of experts certifies brainstem death then the registered medical practitioner of the hospital having ICU facility with the transplant coordinator, if available, will contact the next of kin with required forms and appropriate checks as directed in the Act.

Social and Cultural Dilemmas in Transplantation

India is a multicultural country with many religions and social problems and misconceptions regarding modern medical technology. There are cultural impediments to the donation of body organs. After the death of a loved one, many family members are reluctant to donate organs.

This may happen despite the written permission of the deceased. The main reasons for this are emotional sentiments and the fear of mutilation of body remains. The issue about religion permitting organ donation has been raised in many countries. There are detailed discourses and articles by theologians and ethicists on this topic. Most religions permit living and cadaveric organ donation as this is considered a good deed to save another's life. There are religion-specific resource materials available for the lay public to access and then form own opinion.[19-21]

Allocation of Organs

Another difficult ethical problem to resolve is how to decide who should be given priority to receive deceased organs. Due to the shortage of organs, waiting lists are maintained by the transplant centers in order to rationalize the requirements for prioritization of patients according to the disease severity, medical urgency, and/or life expectancy. Issues on tissue compatibility, blood type, and size are also important as they will impact on the success of transplant. The hospitals should have a board that evaluates each patient for need and suitability as a potential transplant candidate. The evaluating team consists of separate doctors, but may include representatives from the transplant team. This panel may also include a psychiatrist/psychologist and social worker.

Although criteria are defined for efficient allocation of cadaveric organs as per the waiting lists, it can still lead to situations perceived as unjust. Even among ethicists, there is a debate on what constitutes fair allocation.[22,23] This discussion has been well elucidated by the Eurotransplant guidelines.[22,23] While advocates of efficiency (social utilitarianism) focus on doing better with the limited resources, the advocates of justice wish to obtain benefit to the worst off by giving organs to the sickest patients. This unfortunately will lead in many cases to decrease in the survival rates. Defining benefit is controversial because social utilitarianism focuses on the good a transplant might do including the social usefulness of the transplant recipient while medical utilitarianism attempts to determine how much medical benefit the recipient would have, including success of transplant, life extension, and quality of life.[22] Current guidelines approach this dilemma by taking into account the principles of justice (waiting time, urgency, etc.) as well as medical benefit (tissue typing, etc.) in the computerized allocation rules and by also including expert medical opinion (audit process) in prioritizing individual patients on the waiting list.[22,23]

Even though most western countries have well described detailed waiting lists and doctors state that jumping the queue is not possible, the rich and famous can work the system to their advantage and often get preferential treatment, which prompted much debate in the USA. Debates raged when ex United States Vice President Dick Cheney, received a heart transplant at the age of 71 years, even when thousands of younger patients waited in line. Dr Eric Topol, cardiologist at Scripps Health in La Jolla, California wrote on Twitter—*"the ethical issue is not that he had a transplant, but who didn't?"*[24] The now deceased Apple chief executive, Steve Jobs, traveled to Tennessee for a liver transplant, even though he lived in another state.[24] The waiting period for different organs may differ in different regions and those who can afford to travel and pay for the necessary pretransplant evaluation tests can go on multiple waiting lists and can travel to the centers with the shortest waiting list or when an organ is available and can fly in a few hours to reach the transplant center. On the other hand, poorer patients are at a disadvantage, as they cannot afford such expensive treatments and many times insurance companies refuse payment for these procedures.[25] Internationally gender disparity is seen with men more likely than women to receive a kidney or other organs for transplant while most of the donors are women.[26,27]

Deceased kidney transplantation has not reached a high level of awareness among the common man in India. Few donations occur outside large institutes, where the medical teams motivate families to donate organs of brainstem dead individuals. Minors are not allowed to donate solid organs when alive, the only exception being the case of anencephalic babies, whose organs may be donated by the parents.[28] **NOTTO** plays a pivotal role in allocation through training of health personnel, record keeping, tracking, etc.[17,18]

Living Donors

Safety of Living Donors

Donor morbidity is a primary area of concern where psychological and medical sequelae of donations have been raised, and appropriate documentation and care is needed in each case. There are health consequences to donating an organ, with even death of donors in some cases like partial liver donation. The health and economic consequence has been studied in the case of kidney donors.[29]

In India due to the dire shortage of deceased organs, the transplant laws permit the spouse to donate (THOA 1994) resulting in wives being the overwhelming majority of donors. This has been a matter of ethical debate even in the West as there may be concerns about unavoidable family pressure and moral coercion and if the transplant fails the wife may feel guilty and develop psychological problems.[26,27]

Affection and Attachment

The provisions available in Sub Clause (3), Clause 9 of Chapter II of the THOA states "If any donor authorizes the removal of any of his human organs before his death under sub-section (1) of Section 3 for transplantation into the body of such recipient, not being a near relative as is specified by the donor, by reason of affection or attachment toward the recipient or for any other special reasons, such human organ shall not be removed and transplanted without the prior approval of the Authorization Committee". This has led to confusion and was previously misused. The varied interpretations of Sub Clause (3), led to exploitative elements on the word "affection". The debates and discussions were heated and have led to the newer guidelines.[18] The new Gazette notification of Rules 2014 now requires videotaping of the entire interview proceedings. Guidelines to the Authorization Committee clearly state that there should be no tout or middleman with the donor, and the donor has to provide an explanation of why she/he wishes to donate, along with documentary evidence in the form of old photographs. They must provide necessary information about their vocation along with financial statements of the past 3 years. This new requirement removes the ambiguity of the term "affection" and may go some way in preventing the sale of kidneys.

Organ Trafficking/Transplant Tourism

The shortage of deceased donors has led to scandals of organ trafficking and black marketing of organs.[30] Poor persons have been known to sell their kidneys to repay debts, and even more horrific are alleged cases of organs being removed without the knowledge of individuals. The latter is more of a popular fictitious theme for novels, movies, and serials than a reality. However, donors have made these claims when they have not been remunerated as promised. In the USA, knowingly acquiring, receiving or transferring any human organ for human transplantation in exchange for money or other consideration is against the law and punishable with prison time and a fine. The previous lack of stringent laws in many other countries had resulted in transplant tourism by rich foreigners coming to countries such as China, Philippines, and even India. This crisis led to the *Declaration of Istanbul*, which states that organ trafficking and transplant tourism should be prohibited because they violate the principles of equity, justice, and respect for human dignity.[31] The current Indian THOA[17,18] guidelines have been designed to prohibit these unethical practices.

Augmentation of the Organ Pool

With such a shortage of organs, several cases of swapping living donors has been reported in order to obtain the most compatible organs for the patient. In this scenario, the patient receives an organ most compatible to them; this is not a commercial activity as all the donors are family donors.[32] Domino transplant is a method of increasing the donor pool, e.g., a man with cystic fibrosis and pulmonary hypertension received a heart and lung transplant. The heart of the cystic fibrosis patient was transplanted into a woman with end-stage cardiomyopathy.[33] Domino transplants are possible for liver as well, in a condition called familial amyloidotic polyneuropathy, a genetic disease of liver which takes usually three decades to manifest its defective consequences. When this person receives a liver transplant usually around the age of 30 years, the removed liver could be transplanted onto another person, who is not expected to survive >20 years, for instance an elderly person or a person with liver cancer in order to provide better quality of life. This is a method of preventing wastage of any viable organ.[32,33] There should be a thorough evaluation of the organ prior to transplant, to prevent the donation of a defective or a compromised organ.[33] National Human Organ and Tissue Removal and Storage Network has been mandated by the Transplantation of Human Organs (Amendment) Act, 2011, to fill up the gap between "demand" and "supply" as well as "quality assurance" in the availability of various tissues by awareness generation, training of health professionals and developing standard operating procedures (SOPs) for brain dead donors.

Patient Safety (Common to Patients Receiving Cadaver or Living Donor Allografts)

- Since the organs transplanted come from another person (living or cadaveric), the patient safety is important. Care must be taken to ensure no errors occur in tissue typing and evaluation for infection risks is required. Commonly tested infections are to be screened for, e.g., human immunodeficiency virus (HIV), hepatitis B and C, syphilis, cytomegalovirus (CMV), etc.[34]
- In order to reduce rejection of the new organ, many immunosuppressive regimens are used. These are essential for the success of transplant. These medications carry risks of toxicity, increased infections, and predisposition to malignancy.[35] The risk of infections and malignancy varies with different organ transplants. It is important to maintain transparency and report adverse effects. Hence, it is the requirement of the transplant team, to ensure fair reporting of results and side effects to protect the rights of patients.
- A study observed a twofold overall increased risk of cancer, corresponding to an excess absolute risk (EAR) attributable to transplantation of approximately 0.7% per year.[35] The cause may be due to increased infections with oncogenic viruses, or unknown infections. Other contributing factors may be alterations of the immune system, due to immunosuppression, underlying previous medical conditions, or direct drug toxicity. The risk of rejection and other complications should be explained to the patient and the family.
- A national registry to collect data on results of transplant will be beneficial to the patient and families. Organ transplant patients at present need lifelong immunosuppression to maintain the allograft. The ethical principle of justice states that rich and poor must have equal access to all medical treatments. To promote this principle, government assistance is needed to ensure lifelong access to the immuno-suppressive medications and necessary tests, as these are at present not free except in some Government hospitals in India which support lifelong medications for immunosuppression especially for those who cannot afford the expenses involved.

Consent

Informed consent of the donor is essential as there are health consequences to donating organs. Long-term risks must be informed along with counseling, which should be well documented. Usually, a panel of experts is required to assess motives of donation, particularly if donor is not related. In India, since the wives or mothers are frequently donors for organs, though most are voluntary, this does pose questions about coercion or emotional pressure.[26,27]

Recipients too need to be informed about their risks, complications such as rejection, high risk of cancer, and be given realistic expected outcomes in their case. They also need to be informed about follow-up, monitoring and need for medications. The risk of cancer, infections, and other side effects of lifelong immunosuppressive drug therapy is often not understood or explained well.

Several cases have been reported of chronic renal failure patients refusing living donor transplant. They did so, because they did not feel comfortable accepting that someone had to suffer for them.[36]

Summary of Current Ethical Considerations in Organ Transplantation

- Determine accurately the onset of death (brainstem death and heart death) as starting point for organ donation.
- Understanding of persons' perceptions and misconceptions is needed to formulate better awareness materials. Including social and religious leaders in the dialogue is necessary.
- Creating awareness of the applications and laws pertaining to brainstem death and organ donation can encourage deceased organ donations.
- Informed consent from donor, relatives of a deceased donor, and from the patient/recipient.
- Safety of living donors is a priority. This should be monitored periodically.
- Fair and equitable allocation of scarcely available resources due to shortage of donor organs.
- Organ swapping and Domino transplants within this framework can be encouraged.
- National or regional waiting lists should be prepared for fair and equitable distribution of organs.
- Adequate infrastructure should be set-up in all states to handle collection, transportation, and transplantation.
- Minimum standards must be ensured for safety of patients, monitoring, and management of complications. This will decrease the trade involving living organs and reduce the need and any compulsion of living donors to donate.
- The donor should be protected from expenses accruing due to the procedures for transplantation, preferably insurance coverage.
- Research and clinical trials—determining the acceptable balance between risk for the patient and benefit for society.

The Law and Rules Governing Organ Donation and Transplantation in India

Due to unregulated organ transplant and organ trafficking, THOA was passed in 1994. To further enhance the efficacy, relevance, and impact of the Act, an amendment was proposed by the states of Goa, Himachal Pradesh, and West Bengal in 2009. The amendment to the act was passed by the parliament in 2011, and the rules were notified in 2014.

The main provisions of the THOA and the Gazette by the Government of India (March 27, 2014 Gazette of India) outline the rules to be followed in the nonrenewable tissue and organ transplants termed as the Transplantation of Human Organs and Tissues Rules.[17,18] There are some differences between Act of 1994 and subsequent rules passed in 2014 **(Table 2)**.

Kidney Transplantation

Kidneys were among the first organs to be transplanted and the first transplants being performed in 1954. This proved to be a medical breakthrough for patients with chronic renal failure, due to congenital abnormalities, hereditary conditions, diabetes, pyelonephritis, or other renal disorders. In India, the majority of kidney donations are from living-related donors. Deceased donation is a very small number, which is now increasing. The living-related donor donates due to altruism, family motivation, and often financial incentives. In 1995, the news reported a scandal of kidney sales in India, with wide media coverage, and such similar episodes come to the attention of the public frequently, due to the shortage of deceased organs and poor awareness of risks to donors.

The physical and economic consequences of donating a kidney have been studied which led to concerns of health of the donors and their future incapacity to work. In a detailed study,[29] it was found that people who sold their kidneys actually did not benefit from the transaction. Money had been paid for the organ, but often the amount paid was less than what was promised. The donor used the money to pay off debts, so that did not contribute to the wealth of the family. More alarmingly, the study showed the donors had diminished wage earning capacity and long-term effects on health.[29] Donors were not well informed and risked harm to themselves, which is exploitation of the poor to benefit the rich. A study of kidney donors several years after they had donated their kidneys, revealed that if they had known the consequences many would not have sold their organs.[29] In the West, a living donor must be counseled for the risks of donation, and the donation must be for an altruistic reason. A small compensation may be given for undergoing surgery, but no monetary incentive for donating a kidney can be given. All transplants carry risks of complications in the recipient too, though with better experience and expertise many complications and risk of mortality have been reduced. However, infections, rejection (acute or chronic), and risk of developing a malignancy persists in the recipient.

Liver Transplant

The first liver transplant was performed in 1963. With the advent of partial liver transplants, living-related donations have become a reality. Previously only deceased donor liver transplants were possible. Liver donation from a living-related donor poses considerable health hazards. The donor is usually a family member who may feel pressurized to donate because of the desperate condition of the patient.[37,38] The various types of living-related liver transplants are right lobe (makes over 60% of total liver), left liver (40% of liver) for

TABLE 2: Evolution of Indian Transplantation of Human Organs and Tissues Rules (some selected salient and important amendments quoted from the act).[39]

Scope	1994 Act Organs	2014 Rules Organs and tissues
Advisory committee and authority	No advisory committee and lack of definition of competent "authority"	Recommended advisory committee to guide and defined competent "authority"
Informed consent process and pledge	Consent process documentation not clear, pledge not required	Added videotaping of consent process Form 7 for pledge required
Donors	Near relative	Expanded near relative and includes grandchildren, grandparents
Authorization body and registration	Authorization at state level registration for organ retrieval	• Added authorization at hospital level if performing >25 transplants per year • Clarified that registration is not necessary for tissue retrieval
Brain death	By a neurosurgeon/neurologist	• Mandatory for all hospitals with ICUs to report brain death • Constitution of brain death certification board • Procedure simplified and allowed in the event of the non-availability of a neurosurgeon/neurologist, a physician and an anesthetist/intensivist, nominated from a panel already approved by the appropriate authority to declare and they should not be from team removing organ
Counseling and transplant coordinators	Required but not made mandatory	Made mandatory
Penalties and charges for organ retrieval	Less penalties and no charges mentioned	Increased penalty and charges for organ retrieval to NGO/governmental agencies
Medicolegal cases	Mentioned	Clarified
Registries	No mention	National human organs and tissues removal and storage network and national registry for transplant are to be established
Inquiry from the attendants of patient in ICU about organ donation	No mention	There is provision of mandatory inquiry from the attendants of potential donors admitted in ICU and informing them about the option to donate and if they consent to donate, then information communicated to the retrieval center
Swap donation	No mention	Provision of swap donation included
Enucleation of corneas	Not specified	Enucleation of corneas has been permitted by a trained technician
Protection of vulnerable donors	No mention	The Act has made provision of greater caution in case of minors and foreign nationals and prohibition of organ donation from mentally challenged persons

(ICU: intensive care unit; NGO: nongovernmental organization)
Source: Modified from Sahay M. Transplantation of human organs and tissues Act-"Simplified". Indian J Transplant. 2018;12(2):84-9.

adult recipients and left lateral lobe (<30%) liver for pediatric transplants.[40] Good surgical and postoperative skills are a prerequisite to any liver transplant or any transplant program. These requirements have also led to a discussion on minimum facilities required to set-up transplant centers, as it is unethical to allow such complex procedures to be performed without adequate infrastructure and training.[37,38]

The recipient may not be aware of the long-term sequelae of immunosuppression. The risk of malignancy after liver transplantation is higher, especially those transplanted for alcohol-related liver disease and hepatitis C virus infection. The risk of lymphoproliferative disease and cancers of the skin, upper airway, and bowel is also increased.[41] There also may be relapse of the initial disease for which the transplant was performed, e.g., hepatocellular cancer, requiring retransplantation in 10% of patients.[41] Other complications include rejection risk, failure due to hepatic vein thrombosis, biliary complications, and bleeding. The patient may be too desperate to make an informed decision and may be influenced by the transplant team. Hence every effort must be made to obtain informed consent both from the living donor and the patient.

Earlier HIV-positive patients were given a low priority for receiving donor organs, but now with the advent of active retroviral agents, many feel that they will be able to survive several decades with transplant and hence should not be denied treatment.[42] The ethics of giving a liver transplant to an alcoholic has also been debated. Many feel that as the alcoholic is responsible for his condition and may relapse into drinking again and that these patients should be given a lower priority for the deceased organs; which are in short supply for other patients.[43] There may also be a lack of social support and an appropriate home environment to ensure that the transplant recipient is able to comply with her/his lifelong immunosuppression regimen.

The shortage of organs for liver transplant has been a major drawback and sociocultural barriers for organ donation have yet to be surmounted. Additionally, there are logistic issues of organ collection and transportation in India, which have prohibited the transport of organs across the states. Since every patient may not have a living-related liver transplant donor, augmentation of the donor pool is required. There is now a growing interest in engineered organs and xenotransplant organs to expand the number of available donor organs, but at present this is not a feasible option.

Lung and Heart Transplant

The first heart transplant was performed in 1968 and the first heart-lung transplant in 1981. Some patients may require only a heart or a lung transplant; others may need both. The indications for heart transplant are cardiomyopathy, heart valve disease with congestive heart failure, severe coronary artery disease, and severe congenital heart disease. Indications for lung transplants are emphysema, α1 antitrypsin deficiency, cystic fibrosis, bronchiectasis, pulmonary vascular disease, and restrictive lung disease.[44]

Patients of cystic fibrosis and other lung diseases can also receive a living-related single lung transplant from a parent. In one such case, the child received two lungs, one from each parent.[45] In such instances, due to genetic similarity, risk of rejection is lower. Living-related lung donation so far appears to be safe for the donor as none have as yet died from this procedure. Rejection-related issues still need to be addressed and work continues on devising the optimum immunosuppressive drug regimen. Cardiac transplants can be performed with deceased hearts, with appropriate consent from donors prior to their illness or with consent from the relatives. As with other transplants, patients should be informed about the realistic expected outcome in their case. Long-term side effects and risks of infection, cancer, and rejection need to be explained.[45,46]

Bowel Transplants

The first bowel transplant was performed in 1967 and the indications of transplants are short gut syndrome due to trauma, necrotizing enterocolitis, and congenital conditions, e.g., Hirschsprung's disease. Ethically this is both lifesaving and results in improvement of quality of life. Both deceased and living-related bowel transplants have been performed. Issues of consent and long-term risks for the patient and living donor are similar as for other living-related transplants. In the case of a minor patient, the surgeon has to let the parents choose between transplant and lifelong total parenteral nutrition.[47]

Limb Transplant

World over around 110 cases of cadaver hand transplant have been documented so far with <3% rejections. In 2015, doctors at Kochi, Kerala have performed first double hand transplants.[48] This is not a lifesaving procedure. The risk of transplant should be weighed with the benefit of realistic outcome.[49] The social circumstances of the patient should be such that they can afford immunosuppressive medications and the management of the resultant complications. Freely given informed consent to the actual expected improvement in functionality of the transplanted limb should be obtained before the patient agrees to undergo the procedure. The transplanted limb may have severe sensory impairment, putting it at risk for injury. Many times a good prosthesis may be more functional than a transplanted limb. We need to be pragmatic and see the benefit of the transplant on the emotional as well as physical well-being of the patient.

Face Transplant

Once a topic of much debate, this is now becoming accepted by both doctors and the public. Once "Morally objectionable," face transplantation is now seen as "feasible and necessary" procedure.[50] This is again not a lifesaving procedure hence the factors of risk of malignancy, realistic expectations regarding functional improvement, and risks of rejection need to be judiciously explained to the patient. Persons with severe disfigurement, whether due to accidents, burns, cancer, etc. suffer both mentally and socially due to ostracization and are not able to lead a normal life. The success of >25 face transplants performed has led to it becoming a procedure, which is now both feasible and acceptable in such cases.[50] Though there may be significant psychological trauma after a disfiguring accident, the patient's perception of her/himself is also dependent on her/his face and adjusting to a new face after an accident/injury, which may result in a changed or new personality.[50] Pre- and post-transplant psychological support is required. As face transplant becomes more common, how will donor tissues be allocated? Only few families would be willing to donate the face of a deceased loved one, for transplant.

Pancreas Transplant

Though the first pancreas transplant was performed in 1966, it was still considered experimental till the 1990s. Though now it can be performed with an adequate success rate, it requires immunosuppression with all the consequent complications. Due to the shortage of deceased pancreas, xenotransplants and engineered organs from stem cells are undergoing evaluation (both discussed in later sections). Diabetics with end-stage diabetic nephropathy may receive combined pancreas and kidney transplants. Ethical issues are the same as with other transplants regarding consent, organ procurement, and allocation. Due to the shortage of human pancreas and fetal islet cells, porcine islet cells have also been tried. Transplantation of fetal islet cells from a host to the liver of a patient has proved to be technically easier and requires less immunosuppression. The first islet transplant was done in 1974. This is now favored over pancreas transplant.[51]

Cornea Transplants

Cornea transplants have achieved a high level of awareness and success in India, with the National Programme for Control of Blindness (NPCB) and issue of Standards of Eye banking in India (2009) guidelines.[52] This has become socially acceptable and family members are not averse to donate the cornea. The magnanimous feeling of helping a blind person and the relatively minor surgery required, may explain the popularity of this organ donation. Drives to encourage cornea donations have been effective and have led to the establishment of eye banks in many parts of the country.

Skin Transplants

Skin transplant is usually autologous, but has been performed from xenotransplants and temporary allografts. However, with the successful use of artificial skin substitutes, these are not required now. There are fewer ethical issues with regard to corneal and artificial skin transplants.

OTHER NEW TYPES OF TRANSPLANTS

Human fetal brain tissue and neural transplants have been used in certain conditions, though at present without much success. The use of brain tissue is met with some innate repugnance, due to moral and ethical feelings and also due to the risk of prion infections, resulting in its infrequent use in transplant.[53] At present, whole eye transplant and brain transplant are not a reality, in case they do ever become technically feasible, many ethical issues will need to be debated and conflicts unraveled.

Fetal Tissue

Deceased Fetal Tissue and Fetal Embryonic Cell Transplant

These have been tried in conditions such as Parkinson's disease and Huntington's chorea. At present, the only condition in which some success has occurred is fetal thymus transplant in DiGeorge syndrome. Fetal tissues show less antigenicity compared to adult tissues. Only research into fetal tissues is being allowed, until more evidence to support any use at all in humans is available.[54-56] Proper oversight and regulation is necessary and appropriately designed and ethically approved research projects are required, to answer important questions. Precautions are needed to ensure the respectful treatment of the fetal tissue. Also, the age of the fetus has been debated so as to ensure that this tissue is taken before the age at which it will feel pain.[55,57] As fetal tissues are not fully differentiated and adapt easily to receive host signals, it was believed that they will grow and integrate with the host tissues. However, the results of such clinical treatments have had many adverse effects and little or no therapeutic benefit.[58]

Fetal Neural Tissue Transplant

The fetal neural tissue due to its immunological *naivete* is less likely to be rejected. There are many ethical concerns regarding source of this tissue. As the brain controls consciousness, scientists and ethicists have wondered if neural cells transplanted from another source will alter one's identity and consciousness. In a study where dopaminergic neurons from fetal neural tissue were transplanted in patients with Parkinson's disease, there were no altered identity or other problems.[53,58] The biggest concern at present is the alarming numbers of severity of adverse effects reported, such as tumors in the brain, where fetal tissue was injected resulting in hydrocephalus and even death and spinal tumors in a child injected for ataxia telangiectasia. This has led to a moratorium banning its use at present.[58,59]

Summary of Guidelines for Fetal Tissue Research[54-56]

- There should be no research on live aborted fetus.
- Tissue for transplant and research should be obtained from legal or spontaneous abortions.
- The mother's consent must be obtained at the time of abortion for donation of fetal tissue, which is sufficient unless the father objects in writing. In case of incest or rape, the father's objection is of no significance.
- The mother will not dictate as to who shall receive the tissue.
- Anonymity of donor and recipient is to be maintained.
- The transplant requirement will not dictate timing of abortion as the well-being of the mother is of utmost concern. The abortion should be planned solely based on the safety of the mother.
- Those participating in termination of pregnancy will not in anyway, be party to the subsequent usage of the fetal tissue.
- No intact fetus will be kept alive artificially for the purpose of transplant.
- Tissues from aborted fetus can be cultured and banked for use in research or transplantation. If such stored tissue is to be subsequently used for any purpose other than the original objective, a fresh sanction will be obtained from the scientific and ethics committees.

- Cells obtained from fetuses will not be patented for commercial consideration for their subsequent usage.
- Retrieval and transplantation of organs of anencephalic fetus/neonate are ethically permissible only after diagnosis of death is made.
- For transplantation of fetal tissue, the following criteria have to be met:
  - There will be a detailed scientific basis for such transplantation.
  - Animal experiments with appropriate approvals and monitoring by Institutional Animal Ethics Committees (IAECs) as per Committee for the Purpose of Control and Supervision of Experiments on Animals (CPCSEA) Rules (for additional details see Reference 56).

Xenotransplant

Transplantation using organs from animals (xenotransplantation) has been an alternative to human organs and the first successful transplant was performed in 1963–1964, before human organ transplants and chronic dialysis were successful. Transplant across species has many technical, medical, and ethical problems.[60,61] It may be objectionable to certain religious groups, for example porcine organs are not acceptable to followers of Islam and Judaism. The pig and goat are seen as potential donors for humans, as physiologically and size-wise their organs are similar to humans.[62]

Other problems include anti-HLA antibody, anti-pig antibody, and cross reactivity. Transplantation rejection is a major problem, which still needs to be resolved.[62,63] If the rejection factor is controlled, then there is a potential for solving donor organ shortage by xenotransplants. There are, however, drawbacks due to rejection, and better understanding of the biology of tissue tolerance is needed.

Diseases such as acquired immunodeficiency syndrome (AIDS) and severe acute respiratory syndrome (SARS) are transmitted from animals to humans.[63,64] Common zoonotic diseases such as porcine CMV and porcine lymphotropic herpes virus are the other risks. Microbiological screening must be done for over 121 organisms, including 36 species of bacteria, 12 species of fungi, mycoplasma, parasites, and various viruses.[64] Source animals must be reared in a sterile environment and they need to be regularly screened for pathogens.

In India, goat is being avidly researched upon as a source animal, as less religious and social taboos are associated with it. Certain animal rights activists' feel that it is not appropriate to raise animals as organ donors, as they are unable to give consent. Prior to the development of recombinant technology, animals have been used for many years to extract hormones. However, at present xenotransplants are not permitted anywhere in the world and only research on them is being conducted as many barriers still exist.

In the future, advances in stem cell therapy, xenotransplants may preclude the necessity of human organ transplant, and provide alternatives to human organs, which are in short supply. These are areas for public debate and the COVID-19 pandemic will also ensure stringent screening for zoonotic viruses and other pathogens with ability to cross infect species.

CONCLUSION

India is a multi-cultural country, having its population from diverse socioeconomic background. This gives a scope for encountering ethical challenges while being involved with modern medical procedures, such as organ and tissue transplantation. A voluntary consent for tissue or organ donation, either by the living individual or the family members, in case of deceased person, is necessary. The medical team has a moral obligation towards explaining the risks involved with transplantation procedure, both for the donor as well as the recipient. Further, strict enforcement of legal safeguards pertaining to organ or tissue transplantation, can serve as a check for unethical practices and thereby protecting the socially disadvantaged population of the country.

REFERENCES

1. Stroncek D, McCullough J. Safeguarding the long-term health of hematopoietic stem cell donors: a continuous and evolving process to maintain donor safety and trust. Expert Rev Hematol. 2012;5(1):1-3.
2. Pulsipher MA, Chitphakdithai P, Miller JP, Logan BR, King RJ, Rizzo JD, et al. Adverse events among 2408 unrelated donors of peripheral blood stem cells: results of a prospective trial from the National Marrow Donor Program. Blood. 2009;113:3604-11.
3. Naina HV, Pruthi RK, Inwards DJ, Dingli D, Litzow MR, Ansell SM, et al. Low risk of symptomatic venous thromboembolic events during growth factor administration for PBSC mobilization. Bone Marrow Transplant. 2011;46:291-3.
4. Halter J, Kodera Y, Ispizua AU, Greinix HT, Schmitz N, Favre G, et al. Severe events in donors after allogeneic hematopoietic stem cell donation. Haematologica. 2009;94(1):94-101.
5. Duarte RF, Labopin M, Bader P, Basak GW, Bonini C, Chabannon C, et al. Indications for haematopoietic stem cell transplantation for haematological diseases, solid tumours and immune disorders: current practice in Europe, 2019. Bone Marrow Transplant. 2019;54(10):1525-52.
6. Lown RN, Marsh SG, Switzer GE, Latham KA, Madrigal JA, Shaw BE. Ethnicity, length of time on the register and sex predict donor availability at the confirmatory typing stage. Bone Marrow Transplant. 2014;49:525-31.
7. Switzer GE, Bruce JG, Myaskovsky L, DiMartini A, Shellmer D, Confer DL, et al. Race and ethnicity in decisions about unrelated hematopoietic stem cell donation. Blood. 2013;121(8):1469-76.

8. Burgio GR, Locatelli F. Transplant of bone marrow and cord blood hematopoietic stem cells in pediatric practice, revisited according to the fundamental principles of bioethics. Bone Marrow Transplant. 1997;19(12):1163-8.
9. Stevens PE, Pletsch PK. Ethical issues of informed consent: Mothers experience enrolling their children in bone marrow transplantation research. Cancer Nurs. 2002;25(2):81-7.
10. Sorror ML, Maris MB, Storb R, Baron F, Sandmaier BM, Maloney DG, et al. Hematopoietic cell transplantation (HCT)-specific comorbidity index: a new tool for risk assessment before allogeneic HCT. Blood. 2005;106(8):2912-9.
11. Ozdemir ZN, Civriz Bozdağ S. Graft failure after allogeneic hematopoietic stem cell transplantation. Transfus Apher Sci. 2018;57(2):163-7.
12. Weisz V. Psycholegal issues in sibling bone marrow donation. Ethics Behav. 1992;2(3):185-201.
13. Hongeng S, Pakakasama S, Anurathapan U, Andersson B. Haploidentical Hematopoietic Stem Cell Transplantation (Haplo-SCT) with Pre-Transplant Immunosuppression (PTIS) and Post-Transplant Cyclophosphamide (Post-Cy) in Severe Thalassemia: Safe Approach and Excellent Disease Control. Blood. 2014:124(21):2571.
14. Alby N. The child conceived to give life. Bone Marrow Transplant. 1992; (Suppl 1):95-6.
15. Burgio GR, Gluckman E, Locatelli F. Ethical reappraisal of 15 years of cord-blood transplantation. Lancet. 2003;361 (9353):250-2.
16. American Academy of Pediatrics Section on Hematology/Oncology; American Academy of Pediatrics Section on Allergy/Immunology, Lubin BH, Shearer WT. Cord blood banking for potential future transplantation. Pediatrics. 2007;119(1):165-70.
17. Ministry of Health & Family Welfare. (1994 and 2011). Transplantation of Human Organs Act, 1994, No.42 of 1994 (Amendment 2011). [online]. Available from: https://main.mohfw.gov.in/sites/default/files/Act%201994.pdf and https://main.mohfw.gov.in/sites/default/files/THOA-amendment-2011%20%281%29.pdf [Last accessed October, 2021].
18. National Organ and Tissue Transplant Organization, Directorate General of Health Services, Ministry of Health and Family Welfare (2014). Transplantation of Human Organs and Tissues Rules, 2014. New Delhi: Gazette of India; 2014.
19. Robson NZ, Razack AH, Dublin N. Review paper: Organ transplants: ethical, social, and religious issues in a multicultural society. Asia Pac J Public Health. 2010;22(3): 271-8.
20. Akbulut S, Ozer A, Firinci B, Saritas H, Demyati K, Yilmaz S. Attitudes, knowledge levels and behaviors of Islamic religious officials about organ donation in Turkey: National survey study. World J Clin Cases. 2020;8(9):1620-31.
21. Oliver M, Ahmed A, Woywodt A. Donating in good faith or getting into trouble Religion and organ donation revisited. World J Transplant. 2012;2(5):69-73.
22. Adams PL, Cohen DJ, Danovitch GM, Edington RM, Gaston RS, Jacobs CL, et al. The nondirected live-kidney donor: ethical considerations and practice guidelines: A national conference report. Transplantation. 2002;74:582-9.
23. Yuan Y, Gafni A, Russell JD, Ludwin D. Development of a central matching system for the allocation of cadaveric kidneys: a simulation of clinical effectiveness versus equity. Med Decis Making. 1994;14:124-36.
24. Dick Cheney's heart transplant sparks debate: Was he too old? Daily News (The Associated Press). (2012). Health Lifestyle. [online]. Available from: https://www.nydailynews.com/lifestyle/health/dick-cheney-heart-transplant-sparks-debate-old-article-1.1050872 [Last accessed October, 2021].
25. Tilney NL, Guttmann RD, Daar AS, Hoffenberg R, Kennedy I, Lock M, et al. The new chimaera: the industrialization of organ transplantation. International Forum for Transplant Ethics. Transplantation. 2001;71(5):591-3.
26. Mathieson PW, Jolliffe D, Jolliffe R, Dudley CR, Hamilton K, Lear PA. The spouse as a kidney donor: ethically sound? Nephrol Dial Transplant. 1999;14:46-8.
27. Malattiri R, Kumar NK. Gender Disparity in Indian Renal Transplantation. AJOB Empirical Bioethics. 2014;5(3):1-7.
28. Canadian Pediatric Society. Use of anencephalic newborns as organ donors. Paediatr Child Health. 2005;10(6):335-7.
29. Goyal M, Mehta RL, Schneiderman LJ, Sehgal AR. Economic and Health Consequences of selling a Kidney in India. JAMA. 2002;288(13):1589-93.
30. Leitner T, Capitanini L. Market For Black Market Organs Expands: When demand exceeds supply, black market organ sales seen by some as a win-win proposition. Chicago: NBC Chicago; 2014.
31. Delmonico FL. The implications of Istanbul Declaration on organ trafficking and transplant tourism. Curr Opin Organ Transplant. 2009;14(2):116-9.
32. Dar R. Swap and Domino Organ Transplantation Transgressing Socio-Cultural and Political Boundaries. Int J Interdiscip Res Innov. 2015;3(1):84-9.
33. Cochrane AD, Smith JA, Esmore DS. The "domino-donor" operation in heart and lung transplantation. Med J Aust. 1991;155(9):589-93.
34. Centre of Disease Control and Prevention. U.S. Department of Health & Human Services (2019). Donor screening and Testing. [online]. Available from: http://www.cdc.gov/transplantsafety/protecting-patient/screening-testing.html [Last accessed October, 2021].
35. Engels EA, Pfeiffer RM, Fraumeni JF Jr, Kasiske BL, Israni AK, Snyder JJ, et al. Spectrum of cancer risk among US solid organ transplant recipients. JAMA. 2011;306(17):1891-901.
36. Gordon EJ. "They don't have to suffer for me": why dialysis patients refuse offers of living donor kidneys. Med Anthropol Q. 2001;15(2):245-67.
37. Soin AS. Ethical dilemmas in living donor liver transplantation. Issues Med Ethics. 2003;11(4):104-5.
38. Whitington PF. Living donor liver transplantation: Ethical considerations. J Hepatol. 1996;24(5):625-7.
39. Sahay M. Transplantation of human organs and tissues Act-"Simplified". Indian J Transplant. 2018;12(2):84-9.
40. Nadalin S, Bockhorn M, Malagó M, Valentin-Gamazo C, Frilling A, Broelsch CE. Living donor liver transplantation. HPB (Oxford). 2006;8(1):10-21.
41. Desai R, Neuberger J. Donor transmitted and de novo cancer after liver transplantation. World J Gastroenterol. 2014;20(20):6170-9.
42. Halpern SD, Ubel PA, Caplan AL. Solid organ transplantation in HIV-infected patients. N Engl J Med. 2002;347:284-7.

43. Martens W. Do alcoholic liver transplantation candidates merit lower medical priority than non-alcoholic candidates? Transpl Int. 2001;14(3):170-5.
44. Studer SM, Levy RD, McNeil K, Orens JB. Lung transplant outcomes: a review of survival, graft function, physiology, health-related quality of life and cost-effectiveness. Eur Respir J. 2004;24(4):674-85.
45. Tonelli MR. Ethical considerations in the treatment of cystic fibrosis. Curr Opin Pulm Med. 1997;3(6):420-4.
46. Crespo-Leiro MG, Alonso-Pulpón L, Vázquez de Prada JA, Almenar L, Arizón JM, Brossa V, et al. Malignancy after heart transplantation: incidence, prognosis and risk factors. Am J Transplant. 2008;8(5):1031-9.
47. Glover JJ, Caniano DA, Balint J. Ethical challenges in the care of infants with intestinal failure and lifelong total parenteral nutrition. Semin Pediatr Surg. 2001;10(4):230-6.
48. Philip S. (2015). In a rare surgery, Kochi hospital transplants both hands of former Afghan soldier. The Indian Express. [online] Available from: https://indianexpress.com/article/india/india-others/kerala-twin-hand-transplant-succesfully-performed-on-ex-army-captain-from-afghanistan/.
49. Benatar D, Hudson DA. A tale of two novel transplants not done: the ethics of limb allografts. BMJ. 2002;324(7343):971-3.
50. Kiwanuka H, Bueno EM, Diaz-Siso JR, Sisk GC, Lehmann LS, Pomahac B. Evolution of ethical debate on face transplantation. Plast Reconstr Surg. 2013;132(6):1558-68.
51. Bottino R, Trucco M, Balamurugan AN, Starzl TE. Pancreas and islet cell transplantation. Best Pract Res Clin Gastroenterol. 2002;16(3):457-74.
52. Directorate General of Health Services, Ministry of Health & Family Welfare (2009). Standards of Eye Banking in India. [online]. Available from: https://nhm.gujarat.gov.in/Images/pdf/NPCB/Guideline/EyeBank-GuideLines.pdf [Last accessed October, 2021].
53. Burd L, Gregony JM, Kerbeshian J. The brain-mind quiddity: ethical issues in the use of human brain tissue for therapeutic and scientific purposes. J Med Ethics. 1998;24(2):118-22.
54. Lahiry S, Choudhury S, Sinha R, Chatterjee S. The National Guidelines for Stem Cell Research (2017): What academicians need to know? Perspect Clin Res. 2019;10(4):148-54.
55. Indian Council of Medical Research & Department of Biotechnology. ICMR-DBT guidelines on stem cell research and therapy. New Delhi: ICMR & DBT; 2006.
56. Indian Council of Medical Research, Department of Health Research & Department of Biotechnology (2013). National guidelines for stem cell research. [online]. Available from: https://www.ncbs.res.in/sites/default/files/policies/NGSCR%202013.pdf [Last accessed October, 2021].
57. Shorr AF. Abortion and fetal tissue research: some ethical concerns. Fetal Diagn Ther. 1994;9(3):196-203.
58. Folkerth RD, Durso R. Survival and proliferation of non-neural tissues, with obstruction of cerebral ventricles, in a Parkinsonian patient treated with fetal allografts. Neurology. 1996;46(5):1219-25.
59. Amariglio N, Hirshberg A, Scheithauer BW, Cohen Y, Loewenthal R, Trakhtenbrot L, et al. Donor-derived brain tumor following neural stem cell transplantation in an ataxia telangiectasia patient. PLoS Med. 2009;6(2):e1000029.
60. Reemtsma K, McCracken BH, Schlegel JU, Pearl MA, Pearce CW, DeWitt CV, et al. Renal hetero-transplantation in man. Ann Surg. 1964;160(3):384-410.
61. Cooper DK. A brief history of cross-species organ transplantation. Proc (Bayl Univ Med Cent). 2012;25(1):49-57.
62. Appel JZ 3rd, Buhler L, Cooper DK. The pig as a source of cardiac xenografts. J Card. Surg. 2001;16(5):345-56.
63. World Health Organization (2005). Statement from the Xenotransplant Advisory Consultation: Xenotransplant: Hopes and Concerns. [online]. Available from: https://www.who.int/transplantation/XenoEnglish.pdf [Last accessed October, 2021].
64. Kumar G, Tuch BE, Deng YM, Rawlinson WD. Limiting potential infectious risks of transplanting insulin-producing pig cells into humans. Pathology. 2002;34(2):178-84.

Ethical Practices and Guidelines for Animal Experimentation in Biomedical Research

Vasantha Muthuswamy

ABSTRACT

Animal experiments constitute a vital tool of biomedical research, and thus provide a precious service to humanity. It is, therefore, an obligatory responsibility of all the stakeholders to treat animals "humanely" and to adhere to the ethical principles enshrined for animal care and welfare to generate quality scientific data. It is necessary to provide them the basic comforts during their maintenance and experimentation as per existing ethical norms. Animal experimentation is necessary at the current level of knowledge to develop new diagnostics, therapeutics, and medical devices to alleviate suffering of animals and humans from various illnesses. However, efforts to develop alternative methods to animal experimentation should continuously be made so that animal use can become totally redundant in future. Till then, those dealing with animal experiments should be familiar with the existing guidelines and regulations and keep themselves updated on recent developments in the area of animal welfare.

INTRODUCTION

"The entire universe and everything in it, animate and inanimate, is His. Let us not covet anything. Let us treat everything around us reverently, as custodians. We have no charter for dominion. All wealth is common wealth. Let us enjoy but neither hoard nor kill. The humble frog has as much right to live as we."

—**Opening lines of Ishopanishad**

"The greatness of a nation and its moral progress can be judged by the way its animals are treated."

—**Mahatma Gandhi**

HISTORICAL PERSPECTIVE

Scientific experiments involving animals have existed for centuries, but their use became more organized since the development of a modern system of medicines in the 19th century.[1] The traditional systems of medicine in the Asian subcontinent had evolved initially by observing behavior of animals and birds seeking remedies from plants pointing toward a man–animal relationship. Ayurveda was divided into *Pashu* Ayurveda and *Vriksha* Ayurveda. Animal products have been used for therapeutic purposes by the traditional medicine practitioners. Animals were also treated with derivatives from plants, animals, and minerals and observed for their response. This is well documented in the ancient literature written in *Charaka Samhita*.[2] Likewise, *Sushruta Samhita* described the use of internal organs of the dead animals to develop and refine the surgical procedures.[3] In the developed countries, the use of animals in biomedical research is said to date back to the time of Galen, in the 2nd century AD.[4] Local myths ascribe the discovery of narcotic effects of the local beverage Kava (*Piper methysticum*) by Samoans and other local tribes to watching the rats becoming intoxicated or paralyzed after eating the root of the plant. This had happened long before the arrival of the Europeans to this area. Nonetheless, the systematic use of animals in biomedical research began late in the 19th century by Louis Pasteur and Robert Koch to study infectious diseases, such as chickenpox, cholera, and anthrax. Subsequently, animal research played a vital role in the discovery of several antimicrobial agents (e.g., sulfonamides and penicillin) and vaccines (e.g., smallpox and poliomyelitis). These discoveries have led to a marked increase in life expectancy and quality of life for human beings as well as domesticated animals, poultry, etc.

CONTROVERSIES IN ANIMAL EXPERIMENTATION: THE NEVER-ENDING DEBATE

The debate on the exploitation of animals for increasing human race survival is not new. In 1780, the British attorney, Bentham, raised the question of moral regard to animals arguing that if the animals cannot talk, can they be allowed to suffer. Such protests led to the passage of the British Anticruelty Act in 1822 and the establishment of the Royal Society for Prevention of Cruelty to Animals (RSPCA) in

England in 1824.[5,6] This laid the path for the establishment of similar acts and formation of animal protection/liberation societies in many other countries.[7] The earliest pivotal document emphasizing the government to formulate guidelines on ethical animal experimentation also came from England by a British Physiologist, Marshall Hall, in 1831. However, the Protection of Animals Act was enacted only in 1911 in the UK, which is now replaced with Animal Welfare Act, 2006.

Hall's document structured around five principles, which even today form the basis of guidelines developed by various countries regarding animal experimentation.[8]

These five principles are as follows:
1. An experiment should not be performed if simple observations can provide that information.
2. No experiment should be performed without a definite and distinct objective.
3. Experiments should not be needlessly repeated.
4. An experiment should be performed under such circumstances as will secure due observation and attestation of its results.
5. Experiments should be instituted with the least possible infliction of pain to the animal.

Despite many groups having raised the issue of association of animal experimentation with pain and cruelty, it took many years for it to gain a global impact. At the same time, it was also prudent to consider that these animal experiments were vital in scientific advancements and were saving countless human lives. The debate truly gained momentum after the advent of Charles Darwin's Theory of Evolution, which was seen to provide a scientific rationale for using animals to predict probable effects on human beings. Surprisingly for the next few decades, the animal protection movement receded due to the successful development of several important and life-saving medicines and vaccines using animal experiments. Nonetheless, in late 1950s pro-animal movements started stirring again among communities, particularly in the United States of America (USA) and United Kingdom (UK). In response to this, British biologists, Russell and Burch, in 1959 enunciated the principle of the "*3Rs*": Replace, Reduce, Refine—for any kind of research conducted on animals.[9] Later in 1975, Peter Singer in his book, *Animal Liberation*, emphasized that exploitation of animals for personal gain is "speciesism" akin to racism.[10] This had further added fuel to the low-slung enthusiasm of people for animal protection. Some global initiatives also took place in 1956 starting with an international non-governmental and non-profit scientific organization being formed by the name of International Committee for Laboratory Animals (ICLA) **(Table 1)**. This committee was a collaborative project of United Nations Educational, Scientific, and Cultural Organizations (UNESCO), Council for International Organizations of Medical Sciences (CIOMS), and International Union of Biological Sciences (IUBS), with a membership of over 100 countries. They formulated international guidelines on basic ethical principles in animal experimentation and procedures for animal husbandry, experimental procedures, and training of professionals involved in animal care. These guidelines laid highest possible international standards for animal research. ICLA was renamed as International Council for Laboratory Animal Science (ICLAS) in 1979. Subsequently in 2012, the CIOMS in collaboration with ICLAS published guiding principles for biomedical research involving animals.[11] Today animal use for biomedical research and product development is considered to be humane and is highly regulated by various local and national bodies in almost every part of the world and any violation is considered a punishable offence.

EMERGENCE OF ANIMAL ETHICAL GUIDELINES: AN INDIAN PERSPECTIVE

India enacted the animal law as early as 1960 called the "Prevention of Cruelty to Animals Act" for the prevention of cruelty to animals in general, which was later amended in 1982.[12] Section 15(1) of Chapter IV of the Act recommended to establish an Animal Welfare Board under the Ministry of Environment & Forests (MoE&F) which is now renamed as Ministry of Forest, Environment & Climate Change (MoFEC), to further ensure the welfare of the animals. Further, Committee for the Purpose of Control and Supervision of Experiments on Animals (CPCSEA) was established in 1964. However, this committee was dissolved later in 1977. Again after 13 years in 1991, Animal Welfare Board of India (AWBI) recommended to the Ministry to reconstitute CPCSEA with a provision to change its main nominee and other members periodically.[13] Subsequently, from April 2019, it is functioning under the ambit of Ministry of Fisheries, Animal Husbandry, and Dairying. The CPCSEA has time and again issued Gazette Notifications of Rules, in December 1998, 2001, and 2006 by the name of "Breeding of and experiment on Animals (Control) and (Supervision) Rules, with a purpose to accomplish its core objectives."[14,15] The CPCSEA also made it mandatory for every institution in the country having animal experiment facility to register with CPCSEA.[16] It also directs the institutions to constitute an Institutional Animal Ethics Committee (IAEC), whose members are mandated to review, approve, and monitor the experimental work along with ensuring welfare of laboratory animals. At present, there are more than 1,750 registered animal facilities for conducting experiments using animals.

From the perspective of education, University Grants Commission (UGC) instructed various institutions to use alternatives of animal experimentation in anatomy, physiology, zoology, etc., and banned the use of animals for dissection and experimentation in the teaching of pharmacy and life sciences courses both at the undergraduate (UG) and

TABLE 1: Worldwide initiatives for animal protection.

Country	Guideline/Rule/Act introduced	Year of operation	Recommendations
India[12,13,17]	Prevention of Cruelty to Animals (PCA)	1960	To prevent cruelty against animals
	Committee for the Purpose of Control and Supervision of Experiments on Animals (CPCSEA)	1991	To ensure no animal is subjected to unnecessary pain or suffering before, during or after experiments are performed
	Breeding and Experiment Rules	1998/2001/2006 amendments	Mandatory registration of animal facilities used for breeding and experiments
	CPCSEA Guidelines for Laboratory Animal facility	2001/2005	To ensure animal husbandry, animal house facilities and humane care of animals
	Guidelines on the Regulation of Scientific Experiments on Animals	2007	To ensure humane and ethical treatment of animals, while facilitating legitimate scientific research involving experiments on animals
China[18,19]	Statute on Laboratory Animal Administration	1988	Act on breeding, husbandry, quarantine, quality control, and staff qualifications
	Regulation on the Management of Laboratory Animal License System	2001	Application, review, issuance, management and supervision of licenses
	Guideline on Humane Treatment of Laboratory Animals	2006	First broad regulation aligned with other countries (US/EU)
EU[18]	EU Directive 86/609/EEC	1986	Laboratory animal welfare
	EU Directive 2010/63/EU	2010	• Harmonization among EU states • Implementation of the 3Rs • Authorization of projects • Highly specific regulations for Great Apes and nonhuman primates
US[18]	Animal Welfare Act 1	1966	• Developed regulations and standards for the care and use of animals • Licensed animal dealers, mandatory registration of research institutions • Recommended to conduct unannounced inspections
	Institutional Animal Care and Use Committee (IACUC)	1986	• Mandatory approval of research protocol • Adherence to the principles of the 3Rs by the investigator
Japan[18]	Guidelines for Proper Conduct of Animal Experiments	2000	Oversighted by IACUC
UK[5,6]	Royal Society for the Prevention of Cruelty to Animals (RSPCA)	1824	• Charity organization promoting animal welfare • Consolidated different animal welfare legislations/ power of arrest for police
	Protection of Animals Act	1911	Regulates the animal testing, animal sources, housing, and humane killing of animals
	The Animals (Scientific procedures) Act	1986/2013 amendments	Replaced with 2010/63/EU
	Animal Welfare Act	2006	Act to make provision about animal welfare replacing the 1911 Act

postgraduate (PG) levels. Because of difficulties in training with a sudden ban, UGC recommended to constitute a Dissection Monitoring Committees (DMC) to look into the use of animals for both UG and PG programs. Its main objective was to reduce the number of animals dissected in PG courses, ensure usage of only laboratory-bred animals, and demonstration of only one species dissection by the faculty in UG courses.[20] In line with the above recommendations,

Medical Council of India (MCI) in its gazette dated 19 March 2014 notified that, for teaching Physiology and Pharmacology in UG curriculum, computer-assisted models should be utilized as an alternative to animal experiments. Further, MCI has allowed department of Pharmacology to develop skills and training as a part of curriculum for PG courses.[21]

The Indian National Science Academy (INSA) issued "Guidelines for Care and Use of Animals in Scientific Research" in 1992 and revised in 2000, which provided additional information on housing of laboratory animals, physiological parameters of animals, training of staff and proper constitution of IAEC, etc.[22] Subsequently, when CPCSEA published its Guidelines for Laboratory Animals Facility in 2001, it accepted most of the recommendations of INSA Guidelines of 1992 updated in 2000. The Ministry of Environment and Forest, Government of India, had also established the National Institute of Animal Welfare (NIAW) in 1999 at Ballabgarh, Haryana. Its mandate was to organize training programs and workshops in animal research and to create awareness about CPCSEA requirements and guidelines. NIAW also stressed the need to improve animal welfare through training and education on various subjects related to animal welfare including animal management, behavior, and ethics.

SIGNIFICANCE OF ANIMALS IN BIOMEDICAL RESEARCH

Laboratory animals are used for a variety of scientific purposes, including teaching and research.

Basic Research

Studies are conducted to understand the regulation of physiological functions and pathogenesis of the disease process. Both ultimately contribute to the development of newer modalities for diagnosis, treatment, and prevention of diseases in both humans and animals.

Development of New Drugs, Diagnostics or Medical Devices

As on date, the use of animals in screening and developing diagnostic tools and as a pharmacotherapeutic agent is indispensable. During the drug development, the potential drug compounds are subjected to detailed safety, pharmacodynamic (what is the drug doing to the body?), and pharmacokinetic studies (what is the body doing to the drug?) in animals. These studies involve evaluation of new chemical entities for acute, subacute, and chronic toxicity (depending upon expected duration in clinical use). The data is generated in both rodent and a nonrodent species at several dose levels to find the minimum toxic and efficacy dose to ascertain a satisfactory risk–benefit ratio. Teratogenic studies are done if drugs are to be used by women of childbearing age. Mutagenicity and carcinogenicity are tested for drugs requiring prolonged use or those chemically related to known carcinogens.

Advances in Veterinary Sciences

Many of the new introductions in the treatment of human diseases have been equally beneficial in veterinary practice. It was estimated that the vaccines developed against anthrax, rinderpest, swine erysipelas, rabies, and canine distemper have saved several million animals.

Production of Healthcare Products

Animal-derived products including hormones (insulin, posterior pituitary hormones, etc.), biologicals (antibodies, immune sera, vaccines, etc.), suture materials, etc. are extensively used in modern medicine. Continuous efforts have been made to obtain these products by in vitro recombinant technology, animal cell lines, etc., which has reduced the use of animals for the production of many healthcare products.

Nonmedical Uses

Animals are also used for safety evaluation of agrochemicals, food additives, xenobiotics, etc. In 2014, India was first among South Asian countries to amend the Drugs & Cosmetics Act to end cruelty toward animals used to test safety of cosmetics. This mandated the development of non-animal alternative tests that could replace invasive tests on animals. This ban also included the import of cosmetics products tested on animals.[23] Additionally, there have also been protests against the use of animals in defense research for testing new weaponry,[24] space research,[25] cosmetic industry,[23] hazards of tobacco smoking/alcohol,[26] car safety research for accident prevention, etc.

Educational Use

Dissection in classrooms requires a large number of animals and is being phased out gradually and replaced by alternative methods/models, such as computer modeling, simulation, interactive softwares, films, charts, and lifelike models. Animals are also used for the maintenance of a variety of pathogens (viruses, bacteria, protozoa, helminths), cancer cell lines, etc. The efforts are being made to replace these applications gradually with in vitro techniques.

Advances in Surgical Technique and Skills

Open heart surgery took about 20 years of animal studies to be perfected. Transplant studies were initially conducted on animals. Experiments on cats helped to develop the techniques for suturing the vessels of the donor organ to the host tissue. Basic studies on the immune systems of several species, such as rodents, rabbits, and monkeys have led to the development of techniques for histocompatibility matching before organ transplant. Development of new inert materials for prostheses, such as the heart valves and hip replacements, also requires preclinical (animal) studies for screening long-term performance and tolerance.

ANIMAL SPECIES USED IN BIOMEDICAL RESEARCH

The species that have been used for research purposes range from unicellular organisms, such as amoebae to large mammals, such as apes and horses. The animals that can be bred and housed in captivity are preferred since they can be reproduced in required strains and numbers with well-defined unique characteristics.[22]

- The use of in-bred strains of rodents, such as mice, rats, hamsters, and guinea pigs, accounts for >90% of the total animals used in biomedical research.
- The use of large animals, namely dog, cat, sheep, pig, fish, frog, bird, horse, cattle, armadillo, nonhuman primates, etc., together make up <10% of the animals used in research.
- The use of endangered nonmammalian vertebrate species, namely amphibians and birds, etc., has been phased out even for educational purposes.
- Genetically modified/transgenic animals have been developed for screening various xenobiotics for several diseases (immunological and transplantation, obesity, hypertension, and diabetes mellitus). Transgenic animals require expertise in breeding and need special husbandry conditions.[22]

ETHICS OF ANIMAL EXPERIMENTATION AND THE DEVELOPMENT OF "Rs"

The initial resistance from the animal activists toward the animal experiments was focused on animal sufferings rather than the principles and outcomes of the experimentation. As mentioned earlier, many scientists themselves could not deny the argument that animal suffering deserves equal consideration as that of a human being.[10] In 1983, Caplan made an interesting distinction between "moral agents" and "moral objects". Moral agents, such as human beings, are capable of moral choice, and hence can claim certain rights. The moral objects, on the other hand, have no duties, and hence cannot claim any rights. He further emphasized that human beings are morally responsible for moral objects.[27] Therefore, scientists engaged in animal experiments should be accountable for the welfare of the animals before, during, and after the experiment. As mentioned before, Russell and Burch were the first to introduce the principle of the "3Rs": Replace, Reduce, and Refine.[9] These slowly led to genesis of the constitution of Animal Ethics Committee (AEC) globally to review all projects directly and indirectly involving animal experimentation. In India, CPCSEA through the establishment of IAEC aims to ensure that the principal investigator follows and implements the approved national guidelines for the use of experimental animals. Also, IAEC ensures that the concept of 3Rs, that is, reduction, refinement, and replacement is implemented.[28] Moreover, after the introduction of anesthesia and refinements in experimental techniques, it is questionable for the activists to overlook the potential benefits of animal use. Hence, an assumption can be made that if any pain or suffering to the animal is present during the experiment, only then it should be considered equivalent to lack of consent.

The 3Rs are mutually complementary and have become the symbol of global efforts to optimize the use of animals in experimental studies.

Reduction in Numbers

- An important fact is to minimize the repetition of animal experiment and permit it only when necessary for some control experiments or for initial standardization.
- Reducing their number also cuts down on the cost and time to complete the study.
- The use of appropriate study designs and statistical tests may support the use of lesser number of animals.
- A critical review of available data in the literature sometimes helps in minimizing the repetition of experiments and avoiding unnecessary use of large animals. For example, if rats and mice are sensitive to pesticides, there is no need to test the same in dogs.
- *Use of special animal strains:* For safety studies small number of responsive species or transgenic strains that are able to express target receptors or molecules provide more consistent results, and thus indirectly reduce the number of animals required for the study.

Refinement of Procedures

The development of more precise experimental techniques with reduced pain and suffering generates reproducible and harmonized data.

- *Improved advanced techniques*: Implantation of lesser invasive sensors, microelectrodes, modern imaging techniques, etc.
- *New biomarkers*: Invention of various surrogate markers has successfully replaced the painful invasive techniques that enable simultaneous and continuous monitoring of the animal in the comfort of its primary enclosure.
- *Improved experimental designs*: Conduct of pilot study to ensure validity of the entire experiment. Newly developed exposure paradigms in immunotoxicology can accommodate differences in the kinetics of immune maturation between human beings and the test species.
- *Refinements in husbandry conditions*: The physical environment of the home cage and animal rooms is an important factor in optimizing the experimental efficiency of the animals.[28]

Replacement Strategies

Replacement means employment of procedures not requiring the use of specified animal species rather than abandoning animal experiments. Replacement of experimental animal with suitable alternative for the purpose of research, education, and regulatory toxicity studies is the ultimate goal. This is the long-term solution compared to the other "*2Rs*" (i.e., reduction and refinement), which are short-term measures.[29] Replacement alternatives to animal experiments can be grouped into four broad categories:

1. Use of non-animal alternatives, e.g., use of computer-based structure–activity relationship software, computer simulated teaching learning models, etc.
2. Use of in vitro procedures, e.g., isolated perfused organs, isolated tissues, single cell or cell lines, subcellular constituents, etc.
3. Use of lower species of animals, e.g., zebra fish and other marine organisms. Horseshoe crab (*Limulus polyphemus*) is used in Limulus amoebocyte lysate assay, which is well accepted as a replacement for the rabbit pyrogen test by regulatory agencies of most countries.
4. Use of ethical human studies (in vivo) in place of animals, e.g.,
   - Microdosing of novel pharmacologic agents in volunteers. In microdosing studies, humans are injected with very low levels of novel substances, which may not pose them any threat.[30]
   - Use of brain imaging technology as a non-invasive procedure to measure brain activity with high level of precision has replaced invasive tests in monkeys.[31]

In India, CPCSEA has pursued not only the principle of 3Rs but also developed additional "*3Rs*", namely Re-use, Rehabilitation, and Responsibility.[32]

Re-use

It is sequential use of same animal for experiments other than the one where it has been used. They can be re-used in other studies following the permission of IAEC. Re-use can be considered as one of the strategies to reduce the number.

Rehabilitation

This usually concerns larger animals used for experimentation purpose. It is the moral responsibility of the principal investigator to provide care and welfare after their use. India is the first country where CPCSEA released the guidelines for rehabilitation of large animals (equines, dogs, etc.) following their use in the experiment.

Responsibility

It is the overall responsibility of all the stake-holders, namely researchers, institutional heads, EC members, animal house supervisors, keepers, etc., to maintain good animal husbandry conditions and abide by existing guidelines and regulations for animal use. It facilitates good health of the laboratory animals, which enables to generate globally harmonized data. From the perspective of ethics, "Responsibility" is the most important principle.

Some scientists believe that the concept of 3Rs or 6Rs framework takes care of animal welfare and animal husbandry and may not necessarily add any scientific value to the animal research. The implementation of earlier 3Rs has led to insufficient statistical power of the study, negative results, lack of reproducibility of animal data, and less scientific publications advocating early *human* research. Three more guiding principles—robustness, registration, and reporting have been suggested by Daniel Stretch and Ulrich Dirnagl to ensure scientific validity of the experiments.[33] Low statistical power of the studies with fewer animals results in the wastage of research funds, inappropriate clinical research outcomes with unnecessary pain and suffering inflicted on the laboratory animals. Reliable, reproducible, and transparent reporting of animal research is an ethical requirement. Therefore, the review and approval of experimental study protocols as required for research on human would identify the shortcomings of the proposal, and this provides an opportunity to the researcher to make the research more robust.

Nonselective reporting helps the effort further for which the ARRIVE Guidelines, "Animal Research: Reporting of In-Vivo Experiments Guidelines" published in 2010 from the UK are recommended. The guidelines consist of a checklist of the items that should be included in any manuscript that reports in-vivo experiments to ensure a comprehensive and transparent description. They apply to mammals and invertebrates and any area of research using live animal species such as observational research, studies conducted in the field and when animal tissues are used. In 2020, an updated version of the guidelines, ARRIVE 2.0 was released, which clearly describes two sets of requirements of 10 each, the "ARRIVE Essential 10", which constitutes the minimum requirements, and the "Recommended Set", which describes the research context.[34]

CONSTITUTION OF INSTITUTIONAL ANIMAL ETHICS COMMITTEE

A properly constituted Animal Ethics Committee should include representatives from departments involved in animal studies, an expert in veterinary medicine, a scientist with adequate knowledge of protection and safety of animals, and a nominee of the community or an NGO organization involved in animal care. The person-in-charge of the animal facility is usually the convener or member secretary. In India, the Breeding and Experimentation Rules made in 1998 by the CPCSEA have laid down the constitution of the

IAEC, and the standard operating procedures (SOPs) for its functioning were made in 2010. The committee should have a biological scientist, two scientists from different biological disciplines, a veterinarian involved in the care of the animals, the scientist in-charge of the animal facility of the institute, a scientist from outside the institute, a nonscientist socially aware member from outside the institute, and a representative or nominee of the CPCSEA. There is provision for co-option of a specialist while reviewing special projects. Chairperson and member-secretary would be nominated by the institution from amongst the members. The committee should be registered with CPCSEA and the registration number should be displayed at the animal facility. Till now, more than 1,750 IAECs are registered with CPCSEA.

FUNCTIONS OF ANIMAL ETHICS COMMITTEE

The main functions of the committee are as follows:
- To review and approve research projects involving animal experimentation.
- To ensure that a minimum number of animals of appropriate species and quality are being employed and that they do not undergo unnecessary suffering during experimentation.
- To review the skill of the scientists and technicians conducting the experiments and confirm its adequacy.
- To ensure the use of appropriate anesthetic, sedative or analgesic and, if indicated, use of an acceptable method of euthanasia at the termination of the study and appropriate methods of disposal.
- To ensure that the animals are provided proper husbandry, appropriate living condition, and veterinary care.
- To strictly follow the specific SOPs applicable to the concerned IAEC based on the CPCSEA guidelines.
- To conduct a periodic review of the ongoing projects and to terminate a study if there is unnecessary suffering to the animals or if generated data does not warrant further study.

The CPCSEA in India has devised forms for submission of research projects for nonhuman primates and other species of animals. The review application must submit the full experimental protocol. It should include clearly defined objectives; details of experimental procedures and drugs to be used; details of the operative procedure, if any, and postoperative care; hazardous drugs/procedures to be used; and safety procedures for the workers, research animals, and other animals in the facility. In 2018, the Ministry of Environment and Forests had released a Compendium of CPCSEA with all relevant acts, guidelines, forms, and formats related to animal experimentation.[35]

CONCLUSION

As on date, animal experiments are essential for the evaluation of new xenobiotics and to benefit the human and veterinary health. The 3Rs of Russell and Burch were implemented for animal welfare and animal husbandry. Further 3Rs were added by CPCSEA emphasizing the responsibilities of all the stakeholders. As these 6Rs were not addressing the scientific need for animal experimentation, Daniel and Ulrich recently introduced further 3Rs to ensure the scientific validity of animal experimentation. "Rehabilitation" of large animals has been specifically emphasized by the CPCSEA in India. All the institutes involved in animal experimentation must get their animal facilities registered with CPCSEA, follow the ethical norms, and constitute local IAECs to ensure humane and ethical treatment of animals while carrying out legitimate scientific research. The most important ethical aspect is the responsibility of researcher as well as all the stakeholders to ensure that the animals are treated humanely by implementing all the Rs, following the existing guidelines and regulations, and keeping themselves updated on recent developments in the area of animal experimentation and welfare.

ACKNOWLEDGMENT

Late Dr BN Dhawan, Former Director, CSIR–Central Drug Research Institute (CDRI), Lucknow, who contributed towards the first draft of this chapter.

REFERENCES

1. Franco AL, Nogueira MNM, Sousa NGK, Frota MF, Fernandes CMSF, Serra MC. Pesquisa em animais: uma reflexão bioética. Acta Bioeth. 2014;20(2):247-53.
2. Sharma PV. The caraka-tattvapradipika of sivadasa sena. Anc Sci Life. 1990;10(2):79-87.
3. Sharma HS, Sharma HI, Sharma HA. Sushruta-samhita-A critical review Part-1: Historical glimpse. Ayu. 2012; 33(2):167-73.
4. Mahajan RC, Sehgal R. Perspective on alternatives to the use of animals in biomedical research. In: Bhardwaj KR, Purohit DC, Dhawan BN (Eds). Laboratory Animal Ethics and Technology. Lucknow: Central Drug Research Institute; 1990. pp. 14-23.
5. Royal Society for Protection of Animals (1972). The History of the RSPCA. [online] Available from: https://www.animallaw.info/article/history-rspca [Last accessed October, 2021].
6. Speaking of research. Animal research regulations in the UK. [online] Available from: https://speakingofresearch.com/facts/animal-research-regulations-in-the-uk/ [Last accessed October, 2021].
7. Miziara ID, Magalhães ATM, Santos MA, Gomes EF, Oliveira RA. Research ethics in animal models. Braz J Otorhinolaryngol. 2012;78(2):128-31.
8. Zurlo J, Rudacille D, Goldberg AM. Animal experimentation: Ethics and law. Animals and Alternatives in Testing: History, Science, and Ethics. New York: Mary Ann Liebert, Inc.; 1994.
9. Russell WM, Burch RL. The Principles of Humane Experimental Technique. London: Methuen; 1959.
10. Singer P. Animal Liberation. New York: Avon; 1975.
11. Council for International Organizations for Medical Science (CIOMS) and the International Council for Laboratory Animal Science (ICLAS) (2012). [online] International guiding principles for biomedical research involving animals. Available from: https://olaw.nih.gov/sites/default/files/Guiding_Principles_2012.pdf [Last accessed October, 2021].

12. Government of India. Prevention of Cruelty to Animals Act, 1960, amended on 30th July 1982. Act No: 59 of 1960.
13. Pereira S, Veeraraghavan P, Ghosh S, Gandhi M. Animal experimentation and ethics in India: the CPCSEA makes a difference. Altern Lab Anim. 2004;32 Suppl 1B:411-5.
14. Committee for the Purpose of Control and Supervision of Experiments on Animals, Ministry of Fisheries, Animal Husbandry and Dairying, Department of Animal Husbandry and Dairying, Government of India. CPCSEA guidelines for laboratory animal facility. CPCSEA; 2001 updated in 2015.
15. Indian Council of Medical Research. Guidance document on animal experimentation. New Delhi: ICMR; 2006.
16. Muthuswamy V, Kumar V. Specific changes needed in the CPCSEA regulations, Ethics in animal experimentation. Proceedings of the 13th Round Table conference. Ranbaxy Science Foundation; 2004. pp. 99-111.
17. Ministry of Social Justice and Empowerment, Government of India. Breeding and experiments on animals (Control and Supervision) Rules of 1998. Gazette Extraordinary Part II section 3(ii); 15 December 1998, pp. 5–26 and its amendments in 2001 and 2006.
18. Institute of Medicine (US); National Research Council (US). International Animal Research Regulations: Impact on Neuroscience Research: Workshop Summary. Washington (DC): National Academies Press (US); 2012.
19. Kong Q, Qin C. Analysis of current laboratory animal science policies and administration in China. ILAR J. 2009;51(1):e1-e11.
20. University Grants Commission. [online] Guidelines for discontinuation of dissection and animal experimentation in zoology/life sciences in a phased manner. Available from: https://www.ugc.ac.in/pdfnews/6686154_guideline.pdf [Last accessed October, 2021].
21. Medical Council of India (2014). Establishment of Medical College Regulations, 2013 (Amendment), (No.MCI-34(41)/2013-Med./64020). [online] Available from: https://www.egazette.nic.in/WriteReadData/2014/158751.pdf
22. Indian National Science Academy (2000). Guidelines for care and use of animals in scientific research. Revised Edition. [online] Available from: https://moam.info/guidelines-for-care-and-use-of-animals-in-scientific-_59f3ea9d1723dded309d0cbc.html.
23. CDSCO. Drugs and Cosmetics (2nd Amendment) Rules, 2014. 148-C: Prohibition of testing of cosmetics on animals. Drugs and Cosmetics (5th Amendment) Rules, 2014. 135-B: Prohibition of import of cosmetics tested on animals. [online] Available from: https://cdsco.gov.in/opencms/opencms/en/Notifications/Gazette- Notifications/ [Last accessed October, 2021].
24. Rawstorne T (2010). Is it really right to blow up pigs even if it saves our soldiers' lives? [online] Available from: https://www.dailymail.co.uk/news/article-1282357/Is-really-right-blow-pigs-saves-soldiers-lives.html [Last accessed October, 2021].
25. Lawler A. Animal activists target NASA mission. Science. 1996;272(5258):26.
26. Shah N. Smoking experiments on animals. (2016). [online] Available from: https://www.petaasia.com/news/smoking-experiments-on-animals/ [Last accessed October, 2021].
27. Caplan AL. Beastly conduct: ethical issues in animal experimentation. Ann N Y Acad Sci. 1983;406:159-69.
28. Mandal J, Parija SC. Ethics of involving animals in research. Trop Parasitol. 2013;3(1):4-6.
29. Hubrecht RC, Carter E. The 3Rs and humane experimental technique: Implementing change. Animals (Basel). 2019; 9(10):754.
30. Lappin G. The expanding utility of microdosing. Clin Pharmacol Drug Dev. 2015;4(6):401-6.
31. Bailey J, Taylor K. Non-human primates in neuroscience research: The case against its scientific necessity. Altern Lab Anim. 2016;44(1):43-69.
32. Committee for the Purpose of Control and Supervision of Experiments on Animals, Ministry of Fisheries, Animal Husbandry and Dairying, Department of Animal Husbandry and Dairying, Government of India (2020). [online] Guidelines of CPCSEA for reuse/rehabilitation of large animals post experimentation. Available from http://cpcsea.nic.in/WriteReadData/LnPdf/GuidelinesofCPCSEAforReuseRehabilitationofLargeAnimals.pdf [Last accessed October, 2021].
33. Strech D, Dirnagl U. 3Rs missing: animal research without scientific value is unethical. BMJ Open Science. 2019;3: e000035.
34. Percie du Sert N, Hurst V, Ahluwalia A, Alam S, Avey MT, Baker M, et al. The ARRIVE guidelines 2.0: Updated guidelines for reporting animal research. PLoS Biol. 2020;18(7):e3000410.
35. Committee for the Purpose of Control and Supervision of Experiments on Animals, Animal welfare division, Ministry of Environment, Forest and Climate Change, Government of India. Compendium of CPCSEA. New Delhi: Ministry of Environment, Forest and Climate Change; 2018.

Index

A

Acquired immunodeficiency syndrome 5, 91
Acute respiratory syndrome, severe 91
Animal ethical guidelines, emergence of 95
Animal strains, use of special 98
Antiretroviral therapy 60
Assisted reproductive technology 59, 60
    complication of 61
    ethical issues in 59, 64
    religious issues in 64
Autologous bone marrow transplant 83
Autonomy 4, 13
AYUSH Hospital Management Information System 69
Azadirachta indica 76

B

Bacopa monnieri 73
Bernard's principle 2
Bioethics 2, 10
    education and training 10
    history and evolution of codes and guidelines 1
Biological diversity, convention on 57
Biomedical research 2, 23, 98
Biomedicine 67
Blood cells 79
Bone marrow 79, 80, 83
Bowel transplants 89
Brainstem death 84, 87
British Anticruelty Act 94

C

Cadaver organ 84
Cardiomyopathy 86
Carotene and retinol efficacy trial 32
Centella asiatica 73
Charles Darwin's theory 95
Chemical-manufacturing-control 73
Chorionic villus sample 82
Cognitive impairment 44
Cord blood banking 82, 83
Cornea transplants 90
COVID-19 10, 48, 49
    disease 69
    outbreak 19
    pandemic 7, 38, 42, 48, 49, 53, 75, 91
Curcuma longa 76
Cystic fibrosis 86
Cytomegalovirus 86

D

Deoxyribonucleic acid 74
DiGeorge syndrome 90
Disability adjusted life years 42
Domino transplants 86
Donor
    consent 81
    issues 84
    type of 80
Drugs and Cosmetics Rules 74

E

Elective single-embryo transfer 61
Electronic informed consent 19
Embryo 61
    handling and rights 61
Environment Protection Act 74
Epidemiological study
    ethical issues in 30
    methods 30,
Ethical issues 30, 59, 64, 75, 81
    concerns on 55
Ethics 1
    committee 5, 15, 31, 42, 52, 71
    review 38
        committee 5
Extracorporeal membrane oxygenation 27

F

Face transplant 89
Fetal embryonic cell transplant 90
Fetal neural tissue transplant 90
Fetal tissue 90
    research, guidelines for 90
Food supplements directive 70
Foreign Contribution (Regulation) Act 56

G

Gamete
    donation 60, 62
    intrafallopian transfer 60
    posthumous collection of 64
Graft versus host disease 79
Granulocyte-colony stimulating factor 80, 83

H

Haploidentical transplantation 82, 83
Healthcare products, production of 97
Hearing loss 25
Heart
    death 87
    transplant 89
Helsinki declaration 5, 24
Hematopoiesis 79
Hematopoietic stem cell 79, 83
    source, types of 80
    transplantation 79, 81-83
Hepatitis
    B 86
    C 86
Herbal medicines 68
Highly active antiretroviral therapy 60
Hirschsprung's disease 89
Horseshoe crab 99
Human Fertilization and Embryology Act 60
Human fetal brain tissue 90
Human immunodeficiency virus 5, 86
    development of 34
    prevention trials
        ethical considerations in 7
        network 7
Human leukocyte antigen 79, 80, 83
Hyperstimulation 62
Hypertension, pulmonary 86

I

Iatrogenic disorders 70
Implantable embryo 62
In vitro fertilization 60
Infertility 59
    severe male factor 60
Informed consent 21, 27, 31, 76
    concept of 14
    document 55
        components of 15
    form 16
    process 13, 25, 43
    review 20
Intellectual disability 44
Intensive care unit 88
Intracytoplasmic sperm injection 60, 61
Ischemic cardiac muscle 83
Istanbul declaration 86

K

Kantian theories 4
Kidney 87
    transplantation 87

L

Leukemia 25
Limb transplant 89
Limulus polyphemus 99
Liver transplant 87, 89
Living donors, safety of 85

M

Material transfer agreement 52
Medicinal plant unit 72

Index

Medicine, complementary 68
Mental disorders 42
Mental health
   and human rights 45
   issues 42
Mental Healthcare Act 44, 45
Mental illness 42, 44, 46
   diagnosis of 43
Multiple pregnancies 61

N

Neural transplants 90
New Drugs and Clinical Trials Rules 9, 14, 54, 71
Nuremberg code 14, 24

O

Oocyte 59, 62
   donation 62
Organ
   allocation of 84
   pool, augmentation of 86
Organ transplantation 79, 87
   ethical considerations in 79

P

Pancreas transplant 89
Parkinson's disease 90
Penicillin 94
Percutaneous epididymal sperm aspiration 60
Peripheral blood stem cells 79, 80, 83
Person with Disability (Rights of Persons with Disability Act) 44
Piper methysticum 94
Poliomyelitis 94
Polycystic ovarian syndrome 62
Pre-conception and Pre-natal Diagnostic Techniques (Prohibition of Sex Selection) Act 62
Preimplantation genetic testing 62
Protection of Children from Sexual Offences (POCSO) Act 48
Psychotherapy 70

R

Randomized control trial 44, 67
Rauwolfia serpentina 72, 73
Red blood cells 79
Rehabilitation 99, 100
Reproduction
   fundamental right 59
   third-party 62

S

Semen donation 62
Skin transplants 90
Smallpox 94
Solid organ transplantation 84
Sperm
   aspiration, microsurgical epididymal 60
   donation 62
   extraction, microsurgical testicular 60
Spermatozoa 59
Standard operating procedures 10, 15, 86, 100
Stem cell 80
   therapy 91
Sulfonamides 94
Surgical sperm retrieval 61
Surrogacy 60, 63
   altruistic 63
   gestational 63
Syphilis 86

T

Testicular sperm extraction 60
Thalassemia 82
Therapeutic misconception 26
Tissue 84
   transplantation 84
Traditional herbal medicinal products directive 70
Traditional medicine 67, 68
   status of 67
Transplantation of Human Organs Act 84, 86, 87
Trichopus zeylanicus 76

U

Umbilical cord blood 79, 80, 83
   transplant 82, 83
Uterine transplantation 64

V

Veterinary sciences, advances in 97

X

Xenotransplant 91

Z

Zygote intrafallopian transfer 60